COUCH
TO ACTIVE

Let's spread the word!
XOXO!

Lyn Lindbergh

Praise for COUCH to ACTIVE

In a 'wellness' era characterized by magic-bullet gym memberships, expensive training sessions, and even some shaming, it's refreshing to see Lyn's approach! Everyone's circumstances are unique, but the notion of just getting moving—on a realistic path toward a more active life—is important. Lyn gets it!

—**MARK S. PETERSON,** *Co-Founder and GM of Lard Butt LLC (Lard Butt 1K events)*

COUCH to ACTIVE is one of the best programs out there for helping people ditch their sedentary lifestyles and get moving. Lyn's passion for getting America MOVING again leaps off the page. You can't read her work without coming away inspired and motivated to change. What I love most is that her program isn't just a list of dos and don'ts. She encourages her audience to dig deep, think through barriers, relentlessly pursue breakthroughs, and spread the word to those around them. This isn't a prescriptive, one-size-fits-all diet and exercise plan. This is about creating a sustainable lifestyle that's one big part of a life you love.

—**AMY ROSE DAVIS,** *Story Consultant. www.story-junction.com*

Reading Lyn's book is a different kind of experience for those contemplating tackling a self-help book. Her writing feels like a conversation with a friend while sitting on the couch having tea...no wait, while taking a brisk walk around the soccer field during our kids' game. The decline in physical activity is the single greatest public health threat of our lifetimes. Lyn looks at the monumental challenge facing adults attempting to create work-life balance and provides creative and practical solutions in such a natural way. It feels like great advice from a good friend.

—**HARLOW ROBINSON,** *Executive Director of Healthy Futures and Alaska Sports Hall of Fame*

True beginners needing to make a fresh start are underserved by the mainstream fitness industry. COUCH to ACTIVE meets those who have fallen through the cracks where they're at. It speaks to those who are exhausted, those who are overwhelmed, those who are hurting, and those who are sick of regular fitness approaches. As a fitness professional who specializes in core rehabilitation and helping those who aren't ready for the insanity of typical workouts, I'm so delighted to see this book hit the shelves!

—**BETH LEARN,** *Founder and CEO of Fit2B Studio*

I love the message of COUCH to ACTIVE. As a life-long athlete with physical goals still to achieve, I maintain my fitness by prioritizing training time in my daily routine. If just showing up is daunting, Lyn provides sensible advice on how to achieve that goal peeling away the intimidation.

—**ERDEN ERUÇ,** *holder of 15 Guinness World Records and first person to circumnavigate the globe solo by human power. www.erdeneruc.com*

This is the real deal about creating the life you want and deserve. Lyn has done a fantastic job of breaking down the change we desire in bite size pieces that are poignant yet palatable. What I love about COUCH to ACTIVE is the holistic approach it takes to becoming your best self.

—**VIDA BRATTON,** *Founder of Healthy Curves Rock!*

Lyn's approach in COUCH to ACTIVE is completely different from any other book or program out there. She helps her readers create a true habit by helping them through every step of the process. She leads us through overcoming every possible setback and helps prepare us for the hardest part of the journey to living an active lifestyle—making sure we're mentally ready to stick with it. This book is a must read for anyone who wants to get up off the couch, or who has been frustrated by plans in the past that they haven't been able to follow.

—DR. BETH BROMBOSZ, *Author of* Yoga for Runners

Lyn had me at "Do you want to walk?" It was an easy ask that turned into a lifestyle change. I can walk, I can avoid the couch time after a long day of work, I can do this! And I did it…and made it fun…and haven't stopped. My focus on exchanging couch-time for walk-time or bike-time or other exercise-time has evolved. My habits have changed and my attitude about being active is a primary value in my life. A simple walking challenge changed my life! Thanks Lyn!

—KEVIN O'BRIEN, *Completed all November Walking Challenges*

"I believe I am worthy."

That audacious statement may challenge you if, like me, you grew up believing the gender stereotypes, social myths, and unsustainable social expectations ingrained by family and society at large. But it's a bold mantra to embrace!

Lyn shares powerful secrets we've heard before but, for whatever reason, we ignore, scoff at, or simply refuse to accept. With humor, insight, compassion, encouragement, and enthusiasm, she leads you through mental and physical steps to help you achieve a stronger body, improve your health, and enjoy life more.

Warning: The time it takes to get from "COUCH to ACTIVE" will probably take longer than you either want or expect. Living healthy and actively is a journey, not a destination. But, with Lyn as your guide, you'll come to enjoy each step along the way and stay injury-free.

Remember, you're worth it!

—BONNIE PARRISH-KELL, *Publisher and Chief Diva at Slowpoke Divas*

COUCH to ACTIVE makes fitness achievable and accessible for everyone. I love how Lyn motivates her readers to make movement a part of their everyday lives - and create true and sustainable habits that will help them feel their best day in and day out.

—JAMIE KING, *Founder of Fit Approach*

Lyn gets it. She cuts through the hype the fitness industry has filled our minds with and gives clear strategies to help people live an active lifestyle. If you're still sitting on the couch, you've tried grit and you know about willpower, and those strategies have failed you, COUCH to ACTIVE will take you down a new path that leads to a life you love and a healthy lifestyle you will want to stick with for life.

—KIM PEEK, *Founder and Chief Wellness Warrior at Power of Run and host of Power Up Your Performance Podcast*

For bulk book orders:
Contact COUCH to ACTIVE at beawesome@couchtoactive.com

Disclaimer
To reduce the risk of injury, before beginning this or any exercise program, please consult a health-care provider for appropriate exercise prescription and safety precautions. The exercise advice presented is in no way intended as a substitute for medical consultation. This is especially important if you have a history of high blood pressure or heart disease. If you experience chest pain while exercising, stop immediately. If you feel faint, dizzy, or nauseated, stop immediately. Do not start this program if your physician or health-care provider advises against it. The information in this book is for educational purposes only and is designed to be adapted to the unique needs of your life. Do not ignore the advice of your health-care provider or use the information in this book to avoid following your health-care provider's advice.

The use of any information provided in this book is solely at your own risk.

DEDICATION

To my dad, who said I was no good at sports.
I wish you could see me now.

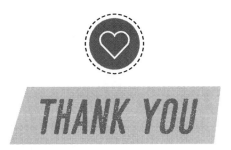

THANK YOU

I'm sitting at my kitchen table watching my puppy Nanu bark at the squirrels, and my heart is overflowing with incredible gratitude for the amazing circle of support that has brought this book to life.

To Amy Rose Davis for carrying all my words with your amazing editing skills: you are not just an incredible editor, you also helped keep me sane and made me a better writer.

To LeAnna Weller Smith and the Weller Smith Design team for your incredible design talent: you stuck with us through all of my perfectionist tendencies and made this work shine. (www.wellersmithdesign.com)

To Tess Oreschnigg for keeping me and this project rolling in the right direction every day and doing it all with a smile.

To Dr. Beth Brombosz for your behind-the-scenes magic that helped me get this book rolling.

To Jim Fagiolo, who did the photography for the cover of the book. I am so grateful that you lent your incredible talent to this work. (www.jimfagiolo.com)

To my mom, Judy, who taught me to believe in myself and gave me an incredible work ethic that has served me well. (Sorry Mom. I promised I'd not mention you in the book; I lied.)

To my hubby, Erik—this book would not exist without your complete moral support and passion for what I do. I am so grateful.

To Amy, Amy, Anne, Anne, Erik, and Erden, for your willingness to share your stories and struggles; your open hearts will most definitely help so many follow your paths.

To all of my clients, who anonymously added to the compilation stories of Jason and Zoe. It has been my honor to serve you.

I also must acknowledge and honor life's struggles. I endured years where my face held a smile, but my heart doubted it would ever feel joy again. I was off-the-charts stressed out and white-knuckling my way through each day. The seven family funerals I attended in three years, the relationships that blew up, and the decade of single-momming it all taught me how to be vulnerable and open my heart to love. The years I cried during my commute to the office, wiping my tears and sucking it up for difficult clients, the Me Too moments I experienced in my own life, the months of being a road warrior for the corporation followed by job loss—these all gave me incredible technical skills and made it crystal clear that life is so much more than the elusive corporate ladder. My stupid asthma that turned out to not be asthma but rather a mystery disease, my fibromyalgia diagnosis, and my migraines all leave me in back of the pack of every sporting event, but they helped me discover the in-the-moment joy of exercise. Holding my father's hand and feeling his slow pulse fade to a flat line taught me how precious life is, and how the only thing that really matters on earth is to love others. Thank you, my dear struggles. Thank you for smacking down my holier-than-thou hyper-functioning dysfunction. Thank you for teaching me how to live a life of humility and compassion for all human beings.

"NO MORE EXERCISE YOU HATE!"

TABLE OF CONTENTS

AT ITS VERY CORE, EXERCISING MEANS:

I believe I am worthy.

I am worthy of health,
I am worthy of strength,
and I am worthy of living a life I love.

Once I figured out that piece,
consistent exercise became easier,
because I was no longer
putting everyone else's whims
before
my
own
health.

I AM WORTHY.

—Lyn Lindbergh

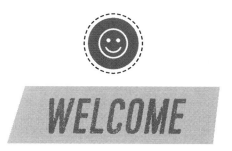

WELCOME

Dear Couch Captive,

You are about find freedom from the almighty power of the couch! Exercise will no longer be one more chore you hate, and getting out the door with your tennis shoes on will not feel like you are trudging through mud. On this journey, you will become a person who exercises consistently and likes it.

No more exercise you hate!

I am not going to teach you how to have more grit, self-discipline, or determination. I won't tell you you're lazy or your priorities are messed up. I know you're not literally slumped over on your couch with your remote, beer, and bag of chips. On the contrary—you are likely a high-performer who is finally taking a look at how to conquer this mission, too.

I used to be there, beating myself up and feeling awful about how hard it was to cram in exercise. I hated how I felt when I didn't exercise, and I hated how I felt when I did. So my stubborn-with-a-smile nature dug in to figure out how to make this work in a way that made me a happier person.

I wanted to thrive as I aged, and I knew that meant I had to include exercise.

I worked relentlessly to figure out the difference between crazy-busy people who exercised regularly and those who consistently struggled. I wanted to figure out how I could get in shape, stay in shape, and still enjoy life. Was this even possible? I was weary of fitness professionals telling me what I needed to do, and I felt like most had no clue about the daily grind I lived. Their recommendations to cram me into what I call "fitness boxes" left me feeling misunderstood and at risk of constant failure. The advice to wake up an hour early to exercise was well-intentioned, but completely lost on me. I was already a sleep-deprived single mom who had to be in a suit and out the door with my child to daycare by 7:15am sharp. My grit and self-discipline were used up on just surviving.

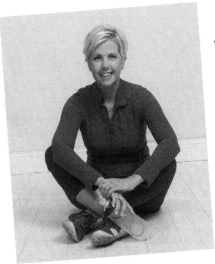

I was massively frustrated. Why is this so hard? What is the gap? It wasn't until years later that I learned my frustration meant I hadn't given up.

I spent over a decade studying and researching the topic. I gained multiple fitness certifications and started teaching fitness classes. In the gym I was seen as a fitness leader, teaching classes with my loud music and over-the-top smile. I was an expert at giving people a great experience.

As I taught fitness classes, I studied my students. I coached people one-on-one and surveyed their lives. I rehabbed people from surgery and mined their experience for what motivated them to keep moving despite major setbacks. I was on a mission to discover behavior themes that the rest of us could learn from.

I wanted to get and stay fit, and I wanted it to be no big deal.

Before I started this journey, I believed that exercise required a super-human level of self-discipline and grit. I needed to just do it, right?

Nope. I was wrong.

I also wrongly assumed that the fit people had cash lying around to throw at memberships and programs to carry them to the finish line. I thought that maybe they didn't have demanding jobs or kids at home, or maybe they didn't have any hobbies or passions. Again—wrong.

Of the people who desire to exercise consistently, why is it that only a few succeed and most fail? If the will to exercise is alive, and you know that exercise is as simple as going for a walk, dancing, swimming, heading to the gym, or hiring a personal trainer, why is it still so hard?

It's hard because getting off the couch is THE hardest exercise of all.

GETTING OFF THE COUCH
IS THE HARDEST EXERCISE OF ALL.

When you conquer the couch, you have won. It's that simple...and that hard!

The piece I found most interesting was that the missing link to getting off the couch has very little to do with exercise plans, workout trackers, or the latest protein powder.

People who have conquered the couch have three practices in common:
They make exercise part of a lifestyle they love.
They adjust with each new phase of life.
They believe they are worth it.

Here's the big mind-blowing concept you need to grasp: **Going from sedentary to active has almost nothing to do with exercise**. Let me say it another way. The things that are keeping you from getting out and doing the exercise you want to do have very little to do with your exercise plans or your gym memberships. We have wrongly assumed that layering gym memberships, programs, and new sports gear on top of our current lifestyle will fix the issue, but it won't. We have to dig deeper than our wallets and discover what is going on in our day-to-day lives.

One day I was out for a long walk and had forgotten my headphones, so I was left with only the thoughts in my head. Everything I had learned over the previous ten years started coming together. COUCH to ACTIVE, that's the missing link! It's a LIFESTYLE change that needs to happen, not another workout program. We need to get our relationships in order. We need to have a strategy for breaking through barriers, and we need to know how to make peace with the barriers that are here to stay. **We need to actually enjoy the exercises we do.**

We need to quit beating ourselves up and start having compassion for where we are today. I had done this for myself and others near me; now I needed to share this gift with the world!

When I got home from that walk, I immediately got cracking on what is now the COUCH to ACTIVE program.

Now it's time for *you* to get rolling!

Sincerely,
Lyn Lindbergh
Your Bad Couch Guru.

P.S. I'm The Bad Couch Guru, because life is more fun with a wink and a smile.

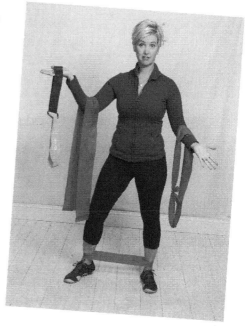

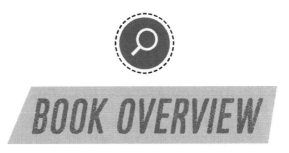

BOOK OVERVIEW

The purpose of the COUCH to ACTIVE program is to look at all of the factors in your life that make it difficult to exercise consistently and make a breakthrough. The hardest exercise you'll ever do is getting off the couch and getting started.

This book is designed to be completed over eight weeks. Don't worry too much about completing it one week at a time. It's more important to focus on completing each lesson and assignment in order.

WEEK 1: The Basics
WEEK 2: Reach Out
WEEK 3: Breaking Barriers
WEEK 4: Solve It
WEEK 5: Own It
WEEK 6: Radical Change
WEEK 7: Your Next Two Years
WEEK 8: Celebrate

👍 **PRO-TIP FOR BOOK CLUBS:** Yes, you can host a book club about exercise while sipping wine! I'm pretty certain you won't be struck by lightning, attacked by a shark, or teleported away by a UFO.

Pitfalls to Avoid

It's no surprise that to get results, you must do the work. This program was originally designed for individuals enrolled in an eight-week coaching program. The live program is highly effective and produces great results. However, a live, in-person format is very limited in the number of people I can reach. I wanted to make this program available to anyone who is motivated. With that said, there are a few pitfalls with having a program like this in a self-study book format.

> **LET'S TAKE A QUICK LOOK AT PITFALLS TO AVOID WHILE WORKING THROUGH THE BOOK.**

Writing in this Book

In order to get the most out of this book, you must have a pen in hand, and you must write in this book. I know this could be especially hard if you are not someone who normally writes in books, so please don't think of this as a book to preserve on your shelf. Your middle school English teacher is not looking over your shoulder anymore. If you want a perfect copy, then buy a second one. Think of this book as your field guide. It will take you toward your new, active lifestyle one step at a time. Life is messy. Let the book join the party.

Speed Reading

This book is designed to be completed over eight weeks. If you must speed read it, go ahead, but then go back and work through the book one week at a time.

Skipping Assignments

The assignments are here for a reason. This book is already the fast track to your active lifestyle. If you rush the process by skipping assignments, the train will derail, and you won't get to your desired destination. Also, many of the lessons refer back to previous assignments.

Criticizing Yourself

Life is crazy-as-bananas, and yours is no exception. If life throws you a curve ball and you fall behind the eight-week schedule, don't beat yourself up. Just pick up where you left off and keep on rolling.

Keeping Momentum

I highly recommend you work though this book with someone to support you. You could work through it with a friend, start your own book club, or sign up for the COUCH to ACTIVE premium program. We can do life alone, but it's so much better with a friend.

Live a Life You Love

If this book doesn't help you love your life more, then what's the point?

WHO ARE JASON AND ZOE?

In addition to sharing my own story, let me introduce you to Jason and Zoe. They will be sharing their stories and tips for applying the lessons in this book.

Jason is a 40-year-old stay-at-home dad. His wife is a partner at a law firm, which means he takes on the responsibility of taking care of the home and their three children. Like many at-home parents, he is so focused on everyone else that the thought of exercising rarely comes to mind. At a recent check-up, his doctor revealed that his cholesterol is high and he's at risk of developing hypertension. He needs to make some changes right away, but the thought of cramming one more thing into days full of kids, chores, errands, and meal preparation is overwhelming and exhausting.

Zoe is a senior manager at a large corporation. She has made a big investment into her career, which is paying off nicely, but she hasn't given her health the attention she knows it needs. She hasn't exercised in years. Now, mid-career, the years of adrenaline and stress with no exercise is taking its toll. Her afternoon double-shot espresso helps her white-knuckle through her daily afternoon energy crash. Most of her evenings consist of takeout for dinner with a glass or so of wine so she can relax. Zoe knows that if she's going to stay on her A-game, she needs to be her best self mentally and physically. But her annual New Year's resolution keeps getting deferred because she hasn't been able to break out of her overly caffeinated, grit-though-at-all-cost habits. She reports to several VPs that seem to be able to stay in shape and wonders why it's so hard for a high-performer like her.

Jason and Zoe are compilations of stories that you will likely be able to relate to. Learn from them both and then decide for yourself how each lesson in this book applies to your unique life.

As you go through every lesson in this book over the next eight weeks, I want you keep one question in the back of your mind the entire time:

HOW CAN THIS HELP ME CREATE A LIFE I LOVE?

This one question is what this book is all about. The active lifestyle you are creating is going to help you live a life you love. Let me say it again: Take every single lesson and ask yourself, "How will this lesson help me live a life I love?"

One of the biggest keys to creating a lifestyle that lasts is to filter every single change to make sure it supports a life you love. If you stay true to this one principle, then you will maintain your active lifestyle, because you will have a life you love more than ever.

Who are all of the other characters?

All of the other stories in this book are real stories from individuals who have shared their stories to help you know that you are not alone and you can conquer significant setbacks and challenges. All of the individuals asked me to use their real names and actual details. This is why so many of the characters are named either Amy or Anne. Those are their real names. Each Amy and Anne story is a different person; it just happened to be a funny coincidence they all had similar names. Thank you Amy, Amy, Erik, Anne, Anne, and Erden for sharing your struggles and hearts with the world! So many will benefit from your willingness to be vulnerable and real.

How Much Exercise?

This book is not specifically about planning and tracking exercise. However, planning and tracking exercise at the start is critical to your success. Your goal is to work toward a lifestyle where you regularly meet the minimum exercise goals recommended by the Centers for Disease Control.

Take a look at the recommendations below. If these recommendations are more exercise than you are currently doing, then spend four to six months slowly working up to this level of activity. As always, consult your physician before starting any new exercise program. You already knew that, didn't you?

The Centers for Disease Control recommend that people focus on two types of exercise: moderate activity and weight bearing exercises.

Minimum Weekly Exercise Recommendation

♡

MODERATE ACTIVITY — 150 minutes

⫟

MUSCLE STRENGTHENING — 2 times

Moderate activity exercise gets your heart pumping. Here are some examples of exercise that fall under the category of moderate activity:

Brisk walk	Biking	Chasing kids	Kick ball
Swimming	Hiking	Power walk the mall	Tennis
Water aerobics	Gardening	Stairs	
Dancing	Duck Duck Goose	Kayaking	
Kick-boxing	Yard work	Surfing	

You'll also want to incorporate muscle strengthening or weight-bearing exercise. This type of exercise will help you build strength and stay injury-free. Many people find it difficult to complete this type of exercise because they think they have to be in a gym lifting weights. Truth is, there are many kinds of muscle strengthening exercises, including:

Weight lifting	Push ups	Calf raises	Back extensions
Yoga	Abdominals	Leg extensions	Modified planks
Pilates	Squats	Bicep curls	
Pull ups		Butterfly press	

RECOMMENDED EXERCISE

Here is one example of how you can follow these exercise recommendations:

♡ = 30 minutes of moderately vigorous activity.

⫼ = Weight-bearing exercise

SUN	MON	TUE	WED	THU	FRI	SAT
♡	♡	⫼	♡	⫼	♡	♡

Don't make the mistake of doing too much, too soon! Start where you are today and add just a little more each week. Do NOT let a personal trainer, friend, or other fitness professional tell you to "go hard or go home." We'll talk more about this message in a future lesson.

Your Assignment

This is your first assignment in our book.

TO-DO	DONE
Find the Weekly Exercise Plans in Appendix C of this book. On Week 1 of the Weekly Exercise Plans, write out your exercise plans for the week. Keep it realistic, and focus on what you would most likely enjoy. It is important that you do not overdo it. Your goal for Week 1 is to simply do a little more exercise than you currently do. If you don't exercise at all, then start with a five-minute daily walk. If you currently hate all exercise, no worries; we'll work on this barrier throughout this book.	✓
In your calendar, schedule your daily exercise for each day of the week.	✓
Send me an email. Include something that is fun or unique about you, or post a picture on social media of you with this book! I want to know what your goals are and what makes you smile! Get creative! Send your email to beawesome@ couchtoactive.com. Include the subject: "(Your Name): My intro."	✓
Find COUCH to ACTIVE on social media and cheer each other on! Bonus points go to pictures of you exercising with the book, dogs, kids, friends, glasses of wine, or steins of beer. Get creative. Our social handle for all is @couchtoactive.	✓

Once you have completed your assignment above, proceed to the next lesson.

If you are not sure where to start with exercise plans, I have a solution for you! The back of this book has a section titled "Exercise Plan Examples" (page 213). These are not your typical exercise plans. They are the simple plans designed to get you started. Don't worry about making a perfect plan for Week 1. Our goal here is to simply have a plan to start with.

Go ahead and take a look at the exercise plan that sounds most like your current situation. Then come back to this page so we can start your journey. This journey is going to be an incredibly valuable experience for you. I'm excited to be your guide!

EXERCISE PLANS:

- I hate exercising, but my doctor is making me do this (page 214)
- My driver's license says I'm 55, but I'll be 30 forever (page 215)

- Help, I just graduated college and am completely out of shape! (page 216)
- I'm a chronic mess of health issues (page 217)
- The baby won't let me sleep! (page 218)
- I hate my asthma! (page 219)
- I seriously need to lose 100 pounds (page 220)
- I dream of doing a marathon (page 221)
- I'm already in great shape (page 222)

Here's an example of what your exercise planners look like:

MY EXERCISE

Create your own exercise plan for the week.

WEEK OF __7__ / __24__ / __18__

TYPE/DAY	EXERCISE	DONE
♡ SUN	*Cardio Walk, 45 min*	✔
♡ MON	*Zumba, 45 min*	◯
⫯⫯ TUE	*Strength Class, 45 min*	✔
♡ WED	*Cardio Walk 45 min*	✔
⫯⫯ THU	*Strength Class 45 min*	◯
♡ FRI	*Roller Blading 45 min*	✔
♡ SAT	*Park Walk 45 min*	◯

Don't forget to introduce yourself!
These emails are the highlight of my week.

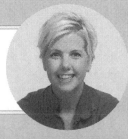

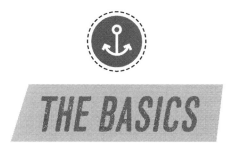

WEEK ONE

What you already know, but aren't doing.

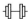

Exercise:

Go to Appendix C of this book and complete your exercise plans for Week 1.

Add your exercise plans to your calendar.

Lessons:

Challenge Your Normal

Call Your Doctor

Injury-free

Remember It

Be a Turtle

Social Media and You

CHALLENGE YOUR NORMAL

Our sense of what is normal for exercise is messed up. Everybody agrees on one thing—that exercise is good for your health. Doctors and scientists all agree on that. We can't even decide if butter is good or bad for us! But when it comes to exercise, it doesn't matter what kind of scientist or doctor you are, your racial or religious identity, or what political views you hold. We all agree on one thing:

EXERCISE IS GOOD.

However, did you know that even though we all agree that exercise is good, there are still about 200 million adults in the United States today who struggle to get the minimum exercise the Centers for Disease Control recommends to help fight many preventable diseases? That's 80% of all adults in the United States, struggling, knowing what we should do, but finding it nearly impossible. Most of us are slowly losing our health. Only 21% of us are getting it right.

WOW.

You are going to change this.

Take a look around you. With only 1 in 5 adults getting the exercise needed, being normal is not good. Exercise is hard because nothing in our lives supports it. Yes, there are gyms, trainers, and an endless number of programs available to us, but most of us have let a gym membership fly by month after month. Our status quo doesn't support it. Life's too busy, work doesn't care, and when we get to the end of our day, the thought of doing the chore of "working out" sounds awful.

Even with all the resources and good intentions, too often, exercise just doesn't happen.

Through this book, I am going to help you make consistent exercise the new normal in your life. Together we are going to make it the new normal in our nation, and we're going to do it all by focusing on living a life you love. Impossible? Not at all.

Today, look around you with these questions in mind.

• *What if exercise were NORMAL for the majority of us?*

• *What if it were NORMAL for everyone to get the exercise they need?*

- *How would YOUR world look different?*

- *How would everything and everyone be different?*

- *What would change?*

- *How much happier would we be?*

- *How much better would you feel?*

- *How would this influence our nation and health-care system as a whole?*

- *Why aren't we there already?*

Imagine yourself going to a corporate retreat where they actually schedule free time for people to exercise, rather than you being the self-righteous freak who crams in a quick workout. It's crazy to me that including this in a multi-day event is currently something only cutting-edge, progressive companies do.

Or imagine an all-day working session where five minutes to stretch each hour wasn't considered a waste of time. Why do we create work environments where the meetings go on for hours, and employees need to sneak away just to use the restroom? Why do we see this martyrdom as a badge of honor? Why do we think this is normal?

If you're not in a desk job, swap these examples above for what you do daily, and the concept still applies. Why have we come to a place as a culture where we make people feel like exercise is a guilty pleasure? Where does this come from?

What if we really did make a shift in our nation? What if we did exercise consistently? How would our moods change? How would our ability to think creatively and solve problems improve? What would the ripple effect be?

Right now, it's easy to feel like getting consistent exercise is impossible and you're somewhat alone in your pursuit of it. But I want to give you a message of hope. You are on the front lines of health and fitness for our nation. Just focusing on meeting the minimum requirements set by the Centers for Disease Control puts you in the top 21% of our nation. By default, you are blazing the trail for greater health and fitness for all. Like it or not, you are a leader!

DID I GET YOU FIRED UP?
GOOD! LET'S DO THIS!

Your Assignment

The purpose of this exercise is to reflect on how the current sedentary lifestyles in our nation have a bigger hold on us than we realize. There are no right or wrong answers on this assignment. Rather, I want you to clearly see your own opinions on this topic.

YOU'LL NEED:

A quiet space where you can think.
A pen or pencil.

WRITE YOUR ANSWER FOR EACH OF THESE QUESTIONS:

1. What would change in your life if exercise were normal for the majority of us?

2. How would YOUR home and work life look different if everyone exercised?

3. How much happier would everyone you interact with be if exercise were normal?

4. How dramatically would the health of our nation improve if we exercised consistently?

5. How would this improvement in the overall health of our nation impact our health-care system?

6. Why is this important?

7. If there are so many benefits, why isn't everyone already exercising consistently?

8. How committed are you to doing your part to create this new normal in yourself?

9. Pause and take a moment to let this all sink in. I find it fascinating how what is normal for exercise doesn't even come remotely close to what the majority of us should do. What are your opinions on the topic?

Congratulations, you have completed your first lesson and are ready to continue to the next lesson.

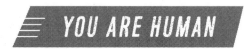
YOU ARE HUMAN

YOU WORK HARD EVERY SINGLE DAY.

Each morning you get up, assess everything you need to do, and do your best to conquer your day. You do your best for your work, and you do your best for your loved ones. Overall, you are rocking it.

This is all fine and dandy, as long as you remember one important fact: you are human. It's easy to get so absorbed with everything we do each day that we forget one very basic fact about ourselves. We forget we are humans, and human beings need to exercise.

My body needs exercise.
My body will always need exercise.
This will never change.
It's not negotiable—it's science.

Pause and slowly re-read the statement above. As you go through life being your usual high-achieving self, there is a lot that will distract you from the simple fact that you are, at your core, a human body. Every single person on the planet, regardless of race, origin, country, language, job, or age needs to exercise. There are absolutely no exceptions. There is no such thing as a super-human who has cracked the genetic code. The zombie apocalypse isn't here, and there's no magic potion or pill that will get you there effort-free. You are a human, and you need to exercise.

It's empowering to pause and remember we're humans because it gives us permission to reprioritize how we spend our days in a way that includes exercise.

We must remind ourselves that exercise is not selfish. It's not a luxury. It's as basic as food, sleep, water, and love.

WE NEED IT. FULL STOP.

We know our bodies need to exercise; this is no surprise. The new habit I want to you to build is to remind yourself, over and over, that exercise is not negotiable. When you are rocking this simple and basic concept, you'll be in a much stronger position to stay motivated.

I make sure to plan out time for my kids to get enough exercise because I know how important it is for their health and that it helps them make good habits for the rest of their lives. But, because I'm so busy taking care of them and household tasks, it was easy for me to forget to get exercise. As caregivers, we need to make sure we're taking care of ourselves! **–Jason**

"MY BODY NEEDS EXERCISE. MY BODY WILL ALWAYS NEED EXERCISE. THIS WILL NEVER CHANGE. IT'S NOT NEGOTIABLE—IT'S SCIENCE."

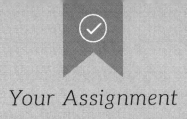

Your Assignment

This is a two-part assignment.

PART ONE: *Memorize it*

1. Write this passage and post it somewhere that you will see it throughout your day.

2. Memorize this so well that you can quote it to anyone in conversation.

I AM HUMAN
My body needs exercise.
My body will always need exercise.
This will never change.
It's not negotiable—it's science.

PART TWO: *Reflections*

REFLECT ON THESE TWO QUESTIONS AND WRITE YOUR RESPONSES BELOW.

1. What would change in your life if you truly believed that exercise was non-negotiable for you?

2. What would change if you truly believed you were worth it?

It's important to quit seeing exercise as a luxury. It's not a luxury at all; it's as necessary to our well-being as eating, sleeping, even breathing! Practice the quote above daily and be able to quote it to me when you meet me someday. Be ready, I'll ask you for it!

Let's move forward to our next lesson.

CALL YOUR DOCTOR

I know that you already know to call your doctor before starting any new exercise program. But this lesson takes an additional angle of how calling your doctor could be exactly the breakthrough you need. Let's unpack this concept further with a story from my life.

I spent years being frustrated with my lack of fitness results. I trained by the book, yet I always landed in the back of the pack. I completed ten triathlons, finished the Seattle-to-Portland 200-mile bicycle ride six times, and survived six half marathons. I ate so healthy that friends teased me; I once actually showed up at a donut fun run dressed up as The Queen of Kale. You could say I was over-the-top driven to perform. Still, I pretty much always finished each event in the back of the pack. I knew this was better than staying home on the couch, but the lack of results was incredibly frustrating. I was living all of the healthy habits, yet my results didn't show it. For a long time, I secretly carried shame about my lack of speed. I felt like such a slowpoke. With no hope of ever placing in a race or ever winning a real trophy, I found myself wondering, "what the heck is wrong with me? What am I doing wrong?"

I HAD TO BECOME MY OWN SCIENTIST AND RELENTLESSLY PURSUE ANSWERS.

My frustration flipped on its head to empowerment when several doctors helped me figure out what was going on with my body. After a year of appointments and tests we discovered that my mild asthma symptoms compromised my fitness a lot more than any of us realized. I discovered I was missing over 30% of my lung function. At the time, I didn't even know I was doing all of this with asthma. I just thought that everyone gasped for air when they ran. I wrongly assumed I was just not trying hard enough.

In addition to medical support, I learned to make one big modification to my exercise habits. I would no longer completely bust my lungs out. I learned how to tell the difference between pushing myself and hurting lungs. When I started to respect my lungs, my whole body started to get stronger.

My health issues will probably always hold me back, and I don't like the fact that I have this lifelong struggle ahead of me. In fact, I spent several years fighting it, doggedly refusing to accept nothing less than complete and total healing. Alas, total healing hasn't been my reality. I will likely always struggle with lung issues. Instead, I have slowly been able to see my health issues as a way to help me have compassion for myself and for others with health issues. In that respect, my health issues that once seemed like a curse to me have become an incredible gift. It helps me reach out to so many others who are also facing their own chronic health struggles. For this, I am grateful.

I still hate being held back and wish there were a magical cure for me. But until that day comes, I have finally quit fighting my health limitations and instead do my best to thrive within my current reality of exercising with health limitations. I have made peace with knowing I will always be a slowpoke, and I have turned my attention toward exercising in a way that brings me joy.

This discovery is worth a lot to me.

Seeking sound medical advice is not a sign of weakness. It's what savvy people do. You are simply gathering more information to make better decisions for your health. With more information about your health, you have more power to do what is right for you!

Please note I am not a medical doctor and am not making any medical recommendations whatsoever. Please do not use my story to make your own medical diagnosis or treatment. Instead, take this lesson as motivation to see your own doctor and get help with any health issues you may be experiencing.

Why This is Important to You: You might be surprised.

It seems as if every person I coach through COUCH to ACTIVE has neglected some medical question or need. I see it so often that I added this lesson because it changes so many lives for the better. For many, it's a complete game-changer.

You must be your own best advocate for your health. Whether you need to see a doctor, naturopath, psychologist, podiatrist, orthopedist, or chiropractor, it is important you recognize that your health is worth it.

YOU ARE WORTH IT.

Getting medical advice isn't a luxury. You are setting the stage for the best health you can give yourself. It is one more step toward finding your strength.

The key takeaway from this lesson is to become committed to your own health. You need to take ownership and make the appointments. You can't wait for a friend, partner, or doctor to tell you what to do. The sooner you own this for yourself, the stronger you will be. Be an example of someone who takes ownership of his or her own health. We need more people like you!

Here I am, looking you in the eyes with a smile, telling you to go call your doctor.

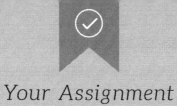

Your Assignment

This is a two-part assignment that could take months or years to fully complete.

PART ONE: *Doctor appointments*

ANSWER THESE QUESTIONS BELOW. BE HONEST WITH YOURSELF.

1. What questions do you have about your physical or mental health?

2. What doctor appointments have you been putting off?

3. Are there modifications to your exercise that you should make to help you accommodate your health needs?

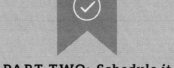

PART TWO: *Schedule it*

TAKE YOUR LIST OF DOCTOR'S APPOINTMENTS YOU HAVE BEEN PUTTING OFF AND SCHEDULE THEM TODAY.

That's right, today. The sooner you get the ball rolling on these, the better.

DOCTOR VISITS TO SCHEDULE

DATE ____ / ____ / ____

ISSUE	DOCTOR TO CALL	DONE

Congratulations! You are on the path to a stronger you.

Now, go make those appointments before you blink and another month flies by!

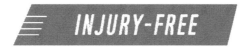

Repeat after me: I am here to heal.

I AM HERE TO HEAL.

I absolutely hated calling home for a bail-out ride when my foot was bothering me on a long walk. When my left knee started "talking to me," I didn't want to slow down on the hills. When my asthma kicked in, I badly wanted to ignore my burning lungs and keep pushing. Pushing through any of these would have caused me injury.

BUT I MADE A PROMISE TO MYSELF.

If it is within my control, injury-free is my decision 100% of the time.

It has paid off. I used to walk about ten miles per week. Now, I'm logging in the ballpark of 30 miles per week. I've slowly and steadily gained strength. I had several rounds of slowing down to avoid injury, but keeping focused on the long-term, avoiding self-inflicted injury, and giving myself time to grow and heal has been the fastest path to progress.

THE TURTLE WINS AGAIN.

Let's be clear. I'm not talking about accidental injuries such as a fall, and I'm definitely not talking about muscles that are sore from working out. I'm talking about overdoing your exercise so much that the effort you are making to become stronger actually hurts you in the long-term.

Why This Is Important to You: You must be compassionate with yourself. Having compassion for ourselves is hard to do.

It's easy to feel like we haven't done enough and should do more. This guilt trap drives us to push harder than we should. The frustration at ourselves, along with being raised with the misguided "no pain, no gain" chant makes anything less than a "go hard or go home" effort feel like a failure. Instead, we need to have compassion for ourselves and start listening to the signals our bodies give us when we are working too hard.

Compassion for ourselves starts with taking a look at how we talk to ourselves. Far too often, our internal self-talk is incredibly toxic, yet we fail to even see it. We go through our day with that voice in our head telling us what we should have done better or should have done differently.

*I absolutely have a Type-A personality. It's been a huge help in the business world, encouraging me to do the hard work that led to many promotions, but it hasn't always served my body well. When I was just out of college, I used to really love running. The thing is, my knee didn't love it. But I'd keep pushing through the discomfort because I wanted to prove to myself that I could push harder and get faster. Finally, my knee had enough, and the pain was so bad I couldn't run anymore. I finally worked up the courage to go to my doctor, who said I had runner's knee. I never did get back into running after that injury, and it spiraled me into years of not exercising at all. The thing is, if I would have taken a couple of days off from running to let my knee heal, I might still be a runner. –**Zoe***

Back before I was aware of my own mysterious health issues, I was terrible at showing myself any compassion. I'd train by the book for a 5K, head to the start line with dread, push through the pain, and finish in the back of the pack. My heart would fill with shame over trying my best and still finishing in the back of the pack. Every. Single. Time. I never gave up, but I always had a cloud of self-doubt and frustration that hung over me. My body wouldn't keep up with my spirit, and I found myself stuffing my anger with a head full of toxic negative self-talk.

I know many of you are already saying, "But wait, Lyn! Don't you hear yourself? You are saying you were ashamed of trying your hardest and doing the best you could with what you had! You should be proud!"

You are right, I should have been proud. But in that moment I hadn't yet learned how to have compassion for myself. It was only after I learned how to be more compassionate to myself that I could then quit making the stupid mistake of pushing to the point of injury. I could face my reality and work with it to the best of my ability. This will never change the fact that I still dream of one day being able to run like a gazelle, but I can now see the bigger picture and realize that finishing first isn't the point, is it?

BY EMBRACING COMPASSION FOR OURSELVES, WE ACTUALLY BECOME STRONGER.

Here are a few examples to help paint the picture of compassion and strength.

"I had a headache this morning and only managed a slow walk for 15 minutes. I'm pathetic." Reframe this negative self-talk to, "I'm glad I moved my body for 15 minutes despite that headache."

....

"That old shoulder injury is acting up, but I'll push through and do my weights." Reframe this to, "It's not worth reinjuring myself. I'll give my shoulder a break and take a walk or do some yoga today."

....

"I feel so fat, ugly, and out-of-shape. I just need work harder, even though my back is killing me. It's the only way I'll get thin." Reframe this horrible self-talk to, "Injury-free IS the fastest path to progress. I'll let my back heal."

....

The takeaway for this lesson is to be committed to gaining strength in a way that is injury-free for you. This will look different for each individual. Your capacity for exercise is unique to you. You only need to be concerned with where you are today.

If you want the fastest path to gain strength and speed, you must commit to paying attention to the cues your body gives you and have compassion for yourself.

The takeaway for this lesson:
Be committed to gaining strength in a way that is injury-free for you.

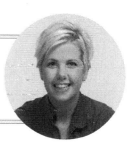

Your Assignment

WRITE YOUR ANSWER TO EACH OF THESE PROMPTS.

1. In what ways have you pushed yourself too hard to the point of causing injury to yourself? This could be physical or mental.

2. Are there adjustments you need to make today to ensure you don't continue to injure yourself?

3. How can you show yourself more compassion?

COMPASSION FOR OURSELVES STARTS WITH TAKING A LOOK AT HOW WE TALK TO OURSELVES.

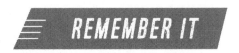

CRUD, I COMPLETELY FORGOT TO EXERCISE THIS WEEK!

We already know that habit is the best way to consistently do something with ease. That's a no-brainer. But when exercise is not yet a habit, thinking about what exercise we will do, when, and with whom, is a lot for the brain to remember. It's easy to go into the day with good intentions about exercising and then simply forget to do it. This alone can make exercise feel like so much work before we even get off the couch.

Simply remembering to exercise can be a barrier to fitness.

You're probably not suffering from early dementia, you don't lack grit, and you're in no way lazy. You're an amazing person who is already doing an excellent job at 100 other things in your life.

WHEN EXERCISE IS NOT CURRENTLY A HABIT, WE NEED TO MAKE IT EASY TO REMEMBER.

Putting the mental chore of remembering to exercise on auto-pilot is one micro-step toward your success. Until this becomes automatic, you'll need help remembering to exercise. You could write a BIG note and put it on your refrigerator or bathroom mirror, set up a calendar invite with a pop-up reminder, or get a dog. Maybe do it all for now! Whatever you choose, figure out what works for you.

CREATE YOUR EXERCISE REMINDERS AND OWN IT!

Continue to have compassion for yourself as you work through the process of remembering to exercise.

Instead of saying "I can't believe I forgot to exercise today! What an idiot! I guess I'll try again tomorrow," reframe your self-talk. "I know it's late, but I can squeeze in 15 minutes of yoga. I'm also going to put a note on my mirror to remind me to exercise tomorrow."

....

Instead of "I got so busy with kids and work that I just put off exercise all day, and now I'm exhausted, and I still have to make dinner," reframe your self-talk as "I got busy with kids and work, but everyone can eat leftovers tonight so that I can do a quick weight workout. I am worthy!"

....

Recognizing that we can easily forget to exercise is a powerful tool. By knowing and admitting how easy it is to forget, we can create a plan to make sure we remember.

TODAY I WILL

(EVERY SINGLE DAY)

EXERCISE PLAN FOR TODAY

WHAT TIME?

WITH FRIENDS?

HOW WILL I REMEMBER?

Here's a pro-tip for my friends. If you have a family calendar, make sure to put your workouts on there! It will be easier to make sure your exercise fits everyone's schedules, and your family members can help keep you accountable, too. —Jason

Your Assignment

PART ONE: *Set reminders*

BELOW IS A LIST OF IDEAS TO HELP YOU REMEMBER TO EXERCISE.

Use this list to help brainstorm your answer to the question below.

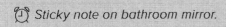

⏰ *Reminder in my calendar.*

⏰ *Alarm on phone.*

⏰ *Sticky note on bathroom mirror.*

⏰ *Big note on kitchen counter.*

⏰ *Note on steering wheel of car.*

⏰ *Set out workout clothes.*

1. What are you going to start doing TODAY to help you remember to exercise every day?

2. Now, go and set up your self-reminders for exercise right now.

PART TWO: *Find your buddies*

Exercise reminders are something you can do completely by yourself. However, a buddy system can also be incredibly powerful.

1. Who in your life could be a buddy who could help you remember to exercise?

2. When will you talk to your friend about helping you remember to exercise?

Most of us will not have instant exercise buddies in place today, and it will take time to find someone. If this is you, then keep your eyes open for someone who can be your support. You will be surprised at how many people out there are hoping to find someone who can help them with their similar journey. Don't be shy! They will be so grateful to find you.

KEEP LOOKING; YOU WILL EVENTUALLY FIND YOUR EXERCISE BUDDIES.

BE A TURTLE

It's hard to be patient, and it's easy to make the mistake of rushing in the name of false progress.

When you aim to make a big change in your life, you can only do it one step at a time. If you rush and force a solution, you are kidding yourself and setting yourself up for disappointment.

This doesn't mean that you are slow and lazy—not at all. You do everything in your power to push through and reach your goals. You take one step, and then you take one more step after that.

WHAT IS YOUR NEXT STEP?

For some of us, our next step is today's exercise. You're actively figuring out how to exercise each day and how to shift other pieces of your life so exercise fits in more naturally. You probably have a few health issues, but nothing that has put your ability to exercise at a complete stand still. Your next step is to stay the course and celebrate each small step.

Some of us, however, have issues we are working through that have put exercise at a complete and full stop. Your next step will be as unique as your current circumstances. If you have health issues preventing any exercise, your next step is to continue to work through your health issues.

 When I first started, I got so overwhelmed by the idea of exercising every single day. I'm already so busy with everything on my to-do list; how could I possibly fit in another thing? The biggest thing that helped me get active was to take things one day at a time. When I looked at the small piece, getting in exercise that day, it was less overwhelming. That mindset shift is what allowed me to finally stick with my active lifestyle. **–Jason**

If you have unique circumstances or hardships making exercise seem impossible, your next step is to be compassionate to yourself. Once you start being kind to yourself, relentlessly pursue how to make your exercise breakthrough.

Have patience when your next step isn't immediately clear. Remember, an unclear path doesn't mean there is no path to your dreams or goals. Your dreams have not been denied. It means you need to keep taking the small steps that are clear until you see the bigger picture.

Stay the course and take it one step at a time.

BE A TURTLE AND YOU WILL WIN.

The takeaway for this lesson:
You are at the beginning of a big adventure. Boil it down to keeping your eyes open and taking it one step at at time. Don't try to conquer it all at once.

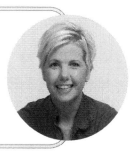

"STAY THE COURSE. ONE STEP AT A TIME. YOU'RE ON YOUR WAY."

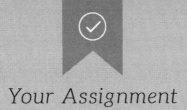

Your Assignment

PART ONE: *Your next five days*

Make a five-day plan of what your next best steps are for your exercise and anything else you need to support this plan. The purpose of this exercise is to think creatively about your next few days and what you can accomplish during this time.

This does NOT have to be perfect. It needs to be simple and realistic.

Here is a sample of what your plan might look like.

ONE STEP AT A TIME

(EVERY SINGLE DAY)

DAY 1 — *Outside walk 30 minutes during lunch. Invite a friend to join me next week.*

DAY 2 — *Walk 30 minutes during kid's game. Talk to kids about needing exercise.*

DAY 3 — *Today is going to be crazy. I'll do 15 minutes of yoga in the morning.*

DAY 4 — *Cycle class at gym. Also, look at gym schedule and see what's new to me.*

DAY 5 — *Yard work with lots of squats. Wash windows with my favorite loud music.*

Get as creative as possible. Today's goal is not to solve the world's exercise problems. Today, we are working to be as consistent as a slow and steady turtle, always moving forward, one step at a time every day.

Challenge yourself to think outside of the box.

If you have a crazy idea to add to your plan that helps you exercise, then yes, you are on the right track.

If you have health issues or unique circumstances that have put exercise at a full stop, then your task is to brainstorm what you are able do in the next five days, no matter how small. It may be micro-session of exercise, like walking for two minutes or stretching. Or, it could be researching more about how you can get back to health.

Most importantly, have compassion for your unique circumstances. You're not alone.

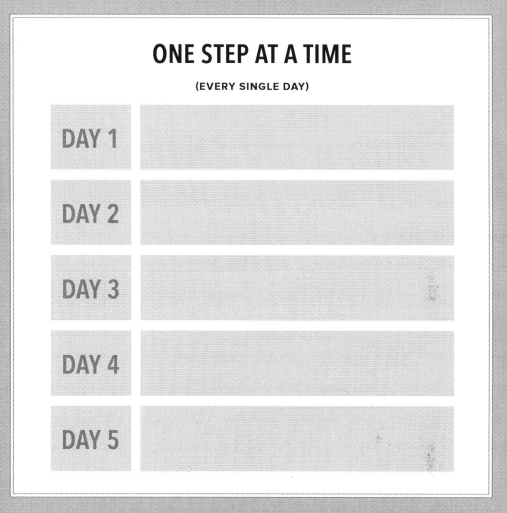

ONE STEP AT A TIME
(EVERY SINGLE DAY)

DAY 1	
DAY 2	
DAY 3	
DAY 4	
DAY 5	

PART TWO: *Your next step*

Pick one of the five items you wrote in the list above and complete the statements below.

1. Right now, my next best step toward exercise is:

2. I will show myself compassion by:

By staying focused on the next step we can take right now, we will stay in action and continue the momentum.

SOCIAL MEDIA AND YOU

SOCIAL MEDIA CAN BE A SOUL-SUCKING SABOTEUR OF OUR SUCCESS. DON'T GIVE IT THAT POWER OVER YOU.

In the second section of this book, Reach Out, we dive into how we can use the social influencers in our lives to help create an active lifestyle. We will look at the real interactions we have with real people in our real lives—not on social media!

Before we get there, I want to take a moment to talk about social media.

We are inundated with messages from every side. Our culture is more media-saturated than ever before. While it's true that we get messages about our bodies from TV, magazines, billboards, radio, and dozens of other media forms, today I want to talk specifically about social media such as Facebook, Instagram, and Twitter.

SOCIAL MEDIA IS A DOUBLE-EDGED SWORD.

On one hand, social media can be a positive and powerful tool for good. It connects people, mobilizes communities, and gives a voice to the unheard. We can use it as a tool to support our goals.

However, we all have experienced how social media can chew us up and spit us out. We feel depressed and anxious by news events, and we find ourselves jealous of our friends' seemingly photo-perfect lives that leave us feeling like a failure.

This is especially true when it comes to exercise. It's so easy to find ourselves back into the negative self-talk of no compassion for ourselves. I know for a fact that I've caught myself hundreds of times in the trap of making assumptions about my friends' social posts that weren't healthy for me.

"Oh, she's such a perfect mom getting out of bed and exercising first thing. Even her sports bra and tennis shoes match! It that 7AM lipstick I see? I'm just over here with coffee and sarcasm." Let's reframe this self-talk to, *"I am just not wired to hop out of bed and exercise first thing, and that's okay. I know I will exercise later because I have my reminders posted."*

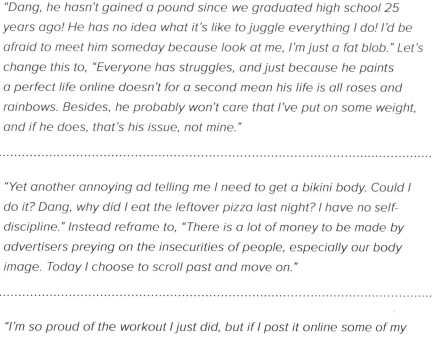

"Dang, he hasn't gained a pound since we graduated high school 25 years ago! He has no idea what it's like to juggle everything I do! I'd be afraid to meet him someday because look at me, I'm just a fat blob." Let's change this to, *"Everyone has struggles, and just because he paints a perfect life online doesn't for a second mean his life is all roses and rainbows. Besides, he probably won't care that I've put on some weight, and if he does, that's his issue, not mine."*

....

"Yet another annoying ad telling me I need to get a bikini body. Could I do it? Dang, why did I eat the leftover pizza last night? I have no self-discipline." Instead reframe to, *"There is a lot of money to be made by advertisers preying on the insecurities of people, especially our body image. Today I choose to scroll past and move on."*

....

"I'm so proud of the workout I just did, but if I post it online some of my friends might mock me or think I'm trying to act better than they are. I'll just keep it to myself." Let's change this to, *"If someone isn't happy about a positive thing I did in my life, that is their issue."*

....

The more you can be aware of what social media does to damage your mindset, the better. As you scroll through your feeds, be hyper-aware of the self-talk you encounter with different types of posts you read.

YOU NEED TAKE OWNERSHIP OF HOW AND WHEN YOU USE SOCIAL MEDIA AND HOW IT HELPS OR HURTS YOUR GOALS.

I personally use social media to help motivate me to meet big goals. This doesn't work for everyone, and it can backfire. It works for me because I know that when I go public with a goal, I have put my ego on the line and am very motivated to get it done just so I can say I did. I'm also not afraid of dealing with a failure online if I don't meet the goal I had made public.

For many of us, using social media to support our goals is not the right decision. There is tremendous social pressure to put our lives online. You don't need to feel that pressure at all. Everyone's social media experience is different, and therefore you should feel empowered to do what is right for you. Own it.

WHY IS THIS IMPORTANT TO YOU?
YOU ARE TAKING OWNERSHIP.

By being aware of how social media impacts your life, you can take ownership of how you use it.

In the following assignment, you will take a closer look at how to ensure social media helps your life goals. You are going to be asked to decide what works for you. You'll need to be decisive.

Let's do this.

Your Assignment

Work through this social media checklist. If you are not on any social media platforms (Facebook, etc.), then do a quick scan of this list and see if any of it applies to other media such as television, magazines, or news media.

TO-DO	DONE
Filter Take a look at the feeds in your social media. If you find yourself anxious, depressed, or jealous after looking at certain pages or people, hide them or unfollow them.	✓
Cheer Others On When someone else posts about exercise, cheer that person on. Exercise can feel like an uphill battle for all of us, and the more we create a culture of supporting each other, the better.	✓
Take Ownership Learn how to use the settings of each of your social media apps. You can turn off most notifications for the social apps so that you aren't constantly bothered by them.	✓
Take Breaks Be conscious about when and how long you are surfing social media and be honest with yourself. Do you need to delete the apps from your phone to limit your time using social media?	✓

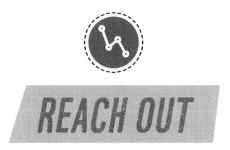

REACH OUT

WEEK TWO

Like it or not, you are now the leader of the pack.

Exercise:

Go to Appendix C of this book and complete your exercise plans for Week 2.

Schedule your exercise plans into your calendar.

Lessons:

Talk

Look them in the Eyes

Reach Out and Lead

Make it Fun

Surprise Them

Thank Them

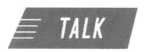

It's time to quit hiding under the cozy blanket on your couch and start talking.

Start talking with everyone in your life about your exercise goals. You'll be amazed at how passionate people are about the role of exercise in their lives, too! When you start sharing what kind of exercise activities you enjoy, others will chime in with energy and ideas. They won't be able to help themselves.

This is an important step in reaching your goals because it transforms how you show up in life. Most of the people around you will be attracted to the newly updated version of you.

The New You:
You are positive, willing to try, and figuring it out.
Keep talking!

Take every opportunity to open up and share your commitment to an active lifestyle. You are no longer going to make it one more chore to cross off the list. No, instead you are making it a new lifestyle. You'll be filling your life with old and new types of exercise you love that bring you to life.

Why This Is Important to You: Words are powerful!

It is true—to some degree, we can talk things into reality. Words are powerful. Talking about your goals out loud, especially to others, helps your brain solidify your goals and intentions. Our brains like to stick with what is familiar. The more you

When I really opened up to my wife about how important my new active lifestyle was to me, the support she gave me was truly incredible. She helped me carve out the time for exercise by helping out with the kids during my workouts. And, she even got my kids in on the support by having them write notes of encouragement that they put on the fridge and in the basement where I do my strength training. I love her so much for this support. ***—Jason***

talk about your new life, the more familiar this will become to your brain. It will make it easier for you to make the transition to an active lifestyle. Without words, your brain will subconsciously try to sabotage your efforts simply because your goals are so unfamiliar.

Don't let this happen.

KEEP TALKING!

As you talk to others about your goals, your brain will shift its mindset. You'll move from "I wish I could be active" to "I am an active person." Once this new idea settles in, your brain will automatically begin to gravitate toward activity. It will begin to because it believes you are an active person. This mindset is powerful and incredibly important.

Start having conversations with the groups below.

GROUP ONE: Your Supporters

Who are the most supportive and encouraging people in your life? Start with these people. Let them know that you're committed to having a fun, active lifestyle. Give them permission to keep you accountable in a way that empowers you and doesn't nag you.

GROUP TWO: Your Friends and Acquaintances

Let your friends know that you're on a mission to figure this out for your life. They will be excited for you. If they also have an active lifestyle, ask them how they do it and see what lessons you can learn from friends who are already where you want to be.

GROUP THREE: Yourself!

How you talk to yourself is critically important. You need to start talking to yourself as if this change is real and has already happened. Here are a few examples of the types of statements you can tell yourself.

- *I am a person who figures out what type of exercise I love.*

- *I am willing to try new things.*

- *I know life will always change, and I love the fact that life never stays the same.*

- *With each new life change, I get creative and adjust my exercise habits.*

- *I always keep trying and searching for ways to exercise that make me smile.*

- *I am not afraid to be super creative, and I don't let so-called experts tell me that my movements are not traditional exercise.*

Let me repeat: Your brain naturally wants to stick with what is familiar and will resist the change you are making. Talking to yourself as if the change has already happened will help fast-track your life change.

> ## "WORDS ARE POWERFUL.
> ## KEEP TALKING."

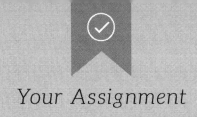

Your Assignment

PART ONE: *Your future is happening today*

Write a paragraph talking to yourself about the active lifestyle you have created as if it already existed today. What does your day look like? What types of exercise are you doing? What new activities have you tried? How do you feel about this change?

PART TWO: *Review daily*

Every day, take a few moments to rehearse the paragraph you wrote above. Think about your new active lifestyle every day as if it is already happening. This will help condition your brain to naturally make this shift in the coming weeks.

Keep talking to yourself every single day as if your new lifestyle is already happening. Keep talking to others to learn, create accountability, and make positive connections.

You are on your way!

LOOK THEM IN THE EYES

This lesson has been my single most powerful tool in finding a way to maintain an active life. Learning this concept was a big deal for me, because I haven't always had this skill or the guts to ask for support from people. Once I finally learned how to advocate for myself in a way that brings people closer to me, magic started to happen. For this, I am forever grateful.

As part of my effort to make exercise a priority, I needed to rally support. I looked people in the eyes and with love said:

> *"My health is important to me, so*
> *I am going make exercise a priority*
> *for the rest of my life*
> *—and I need your support."*

I held that gaze and was amazed at the support I received in return. Of course I received the support, and why was I even surprised? My body needs to exercise, I am worthy of this, and my loved ones recognized it. My close friends were supportive, and I think my husband's exact words were, "You go, girl!"

This isn't a one-and-done conversation. It's not a serious "sit down, we need to talk" discussion, either. Rather, it is a practice of being authentic with each other in

I had been living my new active lifestyle for a few months when I had a deadline for a really big project at work. We all had a lot of work to do, and many of my team members started staying late to keep the project from going sideways. The longer hours made it difficult for me to get in my exercise. I finally came to a breaking point and had to explain to my manager that I needed to get in my exercise. I was vulnerable and told her I have finally been making progress and was afraid I'd slide into a setback if I didn't exercise. Thankfully she was supportive, and I wound up using lunch to get in a daily walk or do some body weight strength training in the office gym. −Zoe

our goals and dreams. It's letting others in your life see your goals and dreams so they can be supportive (or at least be less likely to get in the way). It comes up in our daily light-hearted dialogue around daily plans.

IT IS A LIFELONG PRACTICE.

By showing the strength to ask for support, I am giving my loved ones a clear path to support me and love me.

Looking people in the eyes is important. It ensures you have their attention, and it gives you the opportunity to show them you care with your eyes. They'll see you mean no judgment, you are confident, and you really do want to figure out how to make this a positive experience for both of you.

It's easy to get stuck in a negative cycle of exercise nagging. Our loved ones try to be supportive, but they can come across as judgmental. We want help, but it comes across as a desperate cycle of negative complaining.

Looking them in the eyes with love and compassion puts a stop to all of this.

To some degree, this principle can also be applied to the people you care about at work.

If you come across a complete naysayer, don't worry. We'll address this topic in a future lesson.

"LOOK THEM IN THE EYES. I'M GOING TO MAKE EXERCISE A PRIORITY FOR THE REST OF MY LIFE—AND I NEED YOUR SUPPORT."

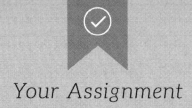

Your Assignment

Talking about having important conversations is good, but if you don't actually start having these conversations, you are not going to see results. In this assignment, you are going to begin having these conversations with your loved ones.

PART ONE: *Eye contact list*

List people in your life who can be your best support. They can be partners, friends, or even your children.

For each person, list how he or she can support you. They could help you carve out time, stay positive, look for activities you enjoy, or simply do their best to not get in your way. Be specific. If you don't know how they can help you, it will be difficult for them to know either.

PART TWO: *Conversations*

Have the conversation with each person in your list. Remember to look them in the eyes.

TIP: DON'T ASK THEM TO NAG YOU. STAY POSITIVE.

Once you have the first conversation, you can mark them as done for the sake of this assignment. Remember, though, this is not a single conversation. It's a new way of communicating daily with the people in your life. It's a new life of supporting each other to exercise and improve our health.

There is a chance you may encounter a neutral or negative response. If this happens to you, don't attach yourself to their positive or negative response. For now, simply have the conversations. In a future lesson, we take a closer look at what to do if you are not met with support.

MY EYE CONTACT LIST

PERSON	SPECIFIC ASK	DONE
My partner	*I will do my best to stay positive. I need him/ her to help me carve out time.*	✓
		✓
		✓
		✓
		✓

REACH OUT AND LEAD

Part of the reason you struggle to exercise consistently is the fact you are a high-performer. That's right, you are awesome at getting things done for other people, and it's one of your greatest strengths.

YOU ARE EXCELLENT AT SERVICE TO OTHERS.

In this lesson, we are going to leverage your ability to serve others in a way that helps you!

Let's take a look at how this concept can play out in your life.

Keep your eyes open and your ears to the ground for others who have similar exercise goals. Remember, 80% of adults in the United States are struggling to get the exercise they need, so finding people with similar exercise goals will be easier than you think. They are everywhere.

It's on everyone's mind. Everywhere I go, the topic of creating an active lifestyle comes up, and I have yet to find a single social situation where anyone truly wants to stay sedentary.

Don't be shy! Share your goals and see if your friends respond with their own similar goals. When they do, bingo! Reach out to them and make an exercise goal. Make the goal as tiny or huge as you like, but most importantly, make it something that will help you both smile.

When you start reaching out to others for exercise-based activities, you are no longer checking exercise off the list of chores for the day—you're living your new active lifestyle!

Thankfully, I have a few co-workers who are also interested in getting in more exercise. We actually started a casual group that is reading this book and trying to exercise more. Office book clubs are rare, and it feels great to help encourage others to get healthy. And even more, the accountability keeps me going. **–Zoe**

"REACH OUT. IT'S NO SECRET THAT IT'S A WHOLE LOT EASIER TO MEET A FRIEND TO EXERCISE THAN TO GO OUT ALONE."

This takes time to build.

There is no quick fix.

Never give up; you will get there.

Why This Is Important to You: Bridges are worth building

This concept is incredibly important. This is where you begin to quit using pure grit and self-discipline to exercise and instead start living a lifestyle where exercise is simply a part of who you are.

Each exercise friendship takes months or even years to build. For the rest of your life, you will be building friendships that include exercise. And since our lives are dynamic and always changing, you'll always be adding new friends to the mix—friends who will help pull you along.

BUT YOU STILL HAVE TO LEAD.

I wish I could tell you that after a few months of leading, your new friends will naturally start returning the favor and inviting you to join them in exercise. Unfortunately, this is an exception to the rule. You will need to be the one who leads and consistently reaches out to others. I have many good friends I have exercised with for over 10 years, and rarely do they extend the invite my way. At first, this reality frustrated me. Why do I have to be the one always carrying the load? But when I relaxed and decided to not let the success of those relationships hinge on whether or not they returned the invites, it got much easier. I didn't let my exercise success depend on whether or not I had a workout buddy, and at the same time I continued to invite people to join me. This landed me in a healthier space where I was in control of my exercise and friends were a positive bonus.

This particular life practice takes years to build and must be rebuilt each time you move to a new city.

This is the beginning of another life practice. When you are open about your goals, you give others the opportunity to join in. When others join, your need for grit and self-discipline nearly vanishes, and you'll build a system of support and encouragement as you become more active.

What do you do if someone doesn't seem interested? It's okay, you're not here to bat a perfect score. In fact, if most of your friends are not interested, don't let this get you down. We have a lot more to cover in this book, and you can succeed at an active lifestyle even if your current friends never join you.

LET'S GET STARTED.

Your Assignment

PART ONE: *Your people*

List the people that you feel comfortable reaching out to today. This is possibly the same list from the previous lesson. The key difference here is that these people won't just encourage you to exercise—they will do the exercise with you. They can be colleagues, friends, or just acquaintances.

  These are people you believe you might be able to exercise with on occasion.

1. _____

2. _____

3. _____

4. _____

5. _____

If your list is short, keep your eyes open for more people to come your way. They are out there; it just takes time to build.

PART TWO: *Make a plan*

When will you reach out to each person on this list? Create a reminder to have each of these conversations.

PART THREE: *Have the conversations*

This may take several weeks, but don't lose track of this assignment! Follow-through is important. These conversations are typically low-key, friendly invitations to exercise. Don't underestimate the power of a simple invite to a friend. The friends who join you will appreciate it.

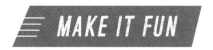

How motivating is it to dread your workout? It's time for you to get radically creative and think of all the possible ways you can make exercise fun. Commit to trying all kinds of exercise until you find a type of exercise you enjoy. To amp up your chances of success, you'll need to let go of stereotypes you have about who does what type of exercise.

IN OTHER WORDS...

NO MORE EXERCISE YOU HATE.

MAKE YOUR EXERCISE FUN—FUN FOR YOU.

It's also time to think outside the traditional exercise box. It doesn't matter if you're working out at the gym with a personal trainer, walking, swimming, dancing with your kids, or taking a fencing lesson. Get creative.

When it's time to plan your exercise for the week, pause and think about what would be the most fun for you. What would make you smile? Do you really want to get on the treadmill again? Or would you rather take the time to walk somewhere beautiful? Do you want to do the same walk for the 100th time? Or maybe tonight, you'll dance in the living room.

Being bold and creative with your exercise will not only make you smile; it will also make the time you spend exercising feel less like a chore and more like a

 Getting active with my kids was a huge game changer for me. We'll all go outside and play freeze tag or kick a soccer ball around. I used to let them go play in the back yard while I did housework or play on the playground while I spent time on my phone or just watched from the edge. Now, I make sure I get active when they get active, too! It's a great bonding experience for all of us—they really enjoy getting to run around with their dad! I don't guilt myself into joining every time. But when I do, I never regret it. **–Jason**

fun activity. You'll be living a life you enjoy rather than counting down the workout minutes left.

Remember, exercise at its core is all about getting the body moving. You don't have to be doing an exact routine to get health benefits. Your body doesn't know the difference between jogging on a treadmill or running from a tiger.

There is now a mountain of research showing that even one minute bursts of exercise are beneficial. I've used this one minute technique on my calves since I was a kid. As a child, I had a few years of ballet lessons where I learned I loved to do calf raises. In ballet, we call it relevé. Long after my childhood ballet days were over, I would still quickly do 50-100 calf raises on a whim. I'd do calf raises standing in line at school, at the grocery store, or brushing my teeth. I've carried this quirky habit with me my entire life. I know, it's a bit odd, and I'll own that. But I find it fun and that's really all that matters, right?

Here's where it gets interesting: I've always had ripped calves, even in my sedentary days. The one minute exercise rule worked.

MOVEMENT IS MOVEMENT. PERIOD.

As you look for ways to add fun exercise into your life, start thinking way outside of the box. If movement is movement, then think of ways you can move your body that are fun. If it either increases your heart rate or adds strength, it counts! That's right, friends, you can have a lot of fun with exercise when you start getting creative.

Why This Is Important to You: Joy matters!

FUN FOR YOU.
NO MORE EXERCISE WE HATE!

Relentlessly pursuing fun exercise not only gives you the energy from exercise, but it also adds a layer of energy from the joy of your activity. This is another piece of magic that will help you create a lifestyle where exercise requires less grit and self-discipline. If you're doing something you enjoy, even the most intense exercise will eventually seem almost effortless.

Think of it this way: the pursuit of fun is critically important to your success. That's right—having fun is a key ingredient of a successful active lifestyle.

Whether you're getting off the couch for the first time in decades or training for your tenth marathon, at the core of your being, you want to live a life you love. Fun will help you get there.

Warning: The Slippery Slope of Exercise Fun

Discovering types of exercise you enjoy is just the beginning. It feels awesome to have the freedom to not cram yourself into a box of fitness and instead just enjoy being active. However, I need to give you a fair warning. As you slowly get in better physical shape, your definition of "fun exercise" is going to evolve. Today you may be going for five-minute walks outside and dancing in your kitchen while nobody is watching. But keep it up, and next thing you know, you'll being leveling up your exercise more and more each month. One month, you might find you actually want to jog a mile. Another month, you might look forward to an exercise class. Be forewarned, because if you blink, you might find yourself far down the slippery slop of exercise fun. Next thing you know, you'll be signing up for a running race or triathlon simply because it sounds like fun! It happens to people who go through this program all the time! Be prepared for the shift. Don't say I didn't warn you. ☺

Your friends and family will notice you relentlessly pursuing FUN exercise. Today, they don't know what to think, but soon they will realize you have said goodbye to the dreaded miserable exercise you hate. They are going to want to join your fun.

 The takeaway for this lesson:
Remember, it's all about living a life you love. Give yourself permission to err on the side of having fun with exercise.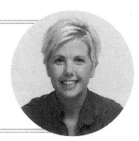

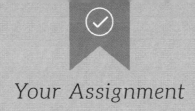

Your Assignment

PART ONE: *Exercise possibilities*

Create these two lists.

LIST #1: FUN EXERCISE

Write down any and every type of exercise that sounds like it could be fun for you. Remember, it's about movement. Get creative.

LIST #2: POSSIBLY FUN IN THE FUTURE

Write down any and every type of exercise that doesn't really sound like fun to you today, but has the potential of being fun in the future when you're in better shape.

Here's an example of the list you are creating.

MAKE IT FUN

YES - FUN	MAYBE - FUN
Weekend dancing	Cycle class
Playing with my child	A 5K run/walk
Sunny day walk	In-home workout
Biking with friends	Personal trainer

Now, create your own list here.

MAKE IT FUN

YES - FUN

MAYBE - FUN

PART TWO: *This week*

Take a look at your two lists. Circle ONE exercise that you can start doing this week. Make a plan right now of when you will start this. Remember, choose only one. You can always go back and do more in the future.

1. What is the exercise you circled in your chart?

2. When will you do this one activity this week?

PART THREE: *Reflections*

1. What will your life look like three months from today if you figure out how to have fun with exercise?

2. Let's imagine you spend the next three months forcing yourself to do exercise you hate. What will your life look like if you ignore the fun factor?

3. How determined are you now to figure out what is fun for you?

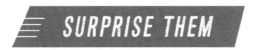

SURPRISE!

You are making a big change in your life, and it's raising eyebrows. It can be especially surprising to those closest to you. If you have tried other programs and failed, your loved ones will be especially surprised when they see you are finally figuring this out. Their surprise is normal. Don't let it throw you off balance.

Those closest to you are accustomed to what has been normal for you. Be it good or bad, they have a picture in their minds of who you are. They haven't fully realized you are making a lasting and permanent change.

YOUR CHANGE IS HERE TO STAY.

It will take time for others to fully realize you have changed.

It usually takes a full three months for those close to you to notice your change at all, and a full year before people in your social circle will actually realize you have changed. That's right—a full year. You'll have many times in that year where you feel the currents of old habits pulling you back into your sedentary life.

By recognizing that it takes months or even years for your social circle to catch on, you can more easily have the strength to stand tall and stick with your change. Your success does not need to be dependent on others recognizing your change.

Here's how this could play out for a holiday.

YEAR ONE: This Thanksgiving, when you go for a walk in the afternoon, it will be a surprise to most of your family and friends, and there's a good chance you'll go alone. You'll still do it and know that this is just the beginning of setting a new routine.

YEAR TWO: Next Thanksgiving, friends and family will arrive wondering if you are going for a walk again (and maybe want to join you). This is where life transformation begins.

YEAR THREE: They arrive expecting the walking tradition. The ship has sailed, and it is now perfectly normal. This is where life transformation has solidified.

Do you see the progression from surprise to normal?

THANKSGIVING EXAMPLE

Year One: Your walk is a surprise.

Year Two: The same friends and family are somewhat expecting it.

Year Three: They expect you will go for a walk.

IT IS A LIFE PRACTICE.

Here are a couple more examples.

THE FRIENDS AND FAMILY CAMPOUT

Year One: Your family is shocked that you did a long hike.

Year Two: Your family wonders if you're going to do a long hike again this year.

Year Three: Your family asks where you'll be hiking this time, because they already know you will.

ANNUAL GIRLS/GUYS WEEKEND

Year One: Your friends tease you for working out daily.

Year Two: Your friends are curious and impressed that you are still working out daily a year later.

Year Three: Your friends expect you will be working out again, and some may even join you!

This is one micro-solution to the larger picture of your active lifestyle. Remember, the accumulation of micro-solutions is what creates an active lifestyle. We'll cover this principle in more detail during week four.

Why This is Important to You: It cultivates patience and resilience. Patience with your social circles is super important. When you realize that your social circles will come around, there is hope. When you understand that this piece takes years to fully settle into place, then you are more likely to have the resilience needed to continue through the years. This is a life practice, and you can find the patience and staying power needed to keep your goals in motion.

IN SHORT: YOU WON'T GIVE UP.

Year One
Surprise them.

Year Two
They expect it.

Year Three
It's perfectly normal.

"SURPRISE THEM OVER AND OVER UNTIL YOUR NEW LIFESTYLE FINALLY FEELS NORMAL."

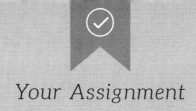

Your Assignment

WRITE YOUR REFLECTIONS TO THE FOLLOWING QUESTIONS:

1. What changes are people seeing in your daily actions today?

2. What additional changes do you want others to see in your actions that they haven't seen yet?

3. What can you do or say that will make it easy for them to support your change?

4. Sometimes friends or family can be intimidated by someone else's positive changes. What can you do or say to assure your friends that you are not judgmental of their sedentary lives?

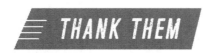

Thank you, thank you very much.

Sometimes the encouragement of well-meaning friends can come across as clumsy, judgmental, critical, and even downright rude. However, what is usually actually happening is they've accidentally fumbled the ball while trying to help you make a touchdown.

Here are a few classic fumbles I see all the time. As you read this list, hear how each statement might be coming from a place of good intention, but can come across horribly.

"Honey, you really SHOULD go exercise."

....

"Just do it."

....

"A marathon runner tells his/her partner that "it just takes discipline."

....

"Would you like a treadmill for your birthday?"

....

"That beer will take 45 minutes to work off."

....

"If exercise were important to you, you'd do it."

....

You're not alone. We've all been there on the wrong side of these fumbles. You know in your head they are only trying to help, but in your heart, it pokes at an area of your life that is particularly sensitive right now. Their encouragement hurts. It leaves you deflated and frustrated, feeling like you're failing at something that should be easier than it is.

Here's the crazy thing: these friends and loved ones sincerely want to help, but they don't know how to help in a way that can also help you both smile. They have the potential to be your best allies if you open up and help them help you. You must be brave, and you must be willing to be vulnerable. Show them how to help.

Here's how to take the misguided encouragement and flip it 180 degrees.

1. Start by thanking them. Even when their encouragement is fumbling, pause and thank them for their good intentions.

2. Give them an example of how they can actually be helpful in a way that would help both of you smile.

You need to figure out what, specifically, your friends can do to support you. If you aren't in touch with what brings you joy, then how could they ever have a chance at getting you there? It must first come from you.

Example for a Friend

> *"Thanks, friend. Yeah, I'm working through this, and I'm committed to figuring out how to exercise more in a way that also creates a life I love. The more we can keep my focus on being positive, the better. How about we go walking together each Wednesday?"*

....

Example for a Partner

> *"Thanks, honey. I really do want to exercise more without feeling like I'm abandoning family responsibilities or sacrificing sleep. Can we brainstorm realistic solutions that could be fun and maybe even make us laugh together a little more? I love you for watching out for me."*

....

Why This Is Important to You: You need positive support.

It's important to thank people—even when their encouragement is clumsy—because it clears the lines of communication. You are rising above the unintended criticism and helping your friends realize that you see their helpful intentions.

By rising above and bringing the conversation to a positive space, it not only improves your relationship with that person, but it'll also help you foster the positive support that will encourage you rather than annoy you.

Note: Sometimes people are just jerks. We'll cover that issue in the "Solve It" section of the book.

Your Assignment

PART ONE: *Your people*

List the people who could be your best allies. Who is trying to help you? This list will probably look similar to your previous lists. The difference between this and other lists is that these are the people you communicate with regularly on a personal level or people who have encouraged you to exercise.

1. _____

2. _____

3. _____

4. _____

5. _____

PART TWO: *Thank them*

This week, proactively thank each person in your list for his or her efforts at being supportive. And then, with as much positivity as you can muster, help them understand how they can be supportive in a way that helps both of you smile.

"Here's how you can help..."

"I don't have it all figured out, but you can help me stay focused on being positive."

"I'm working on living a life I love, and I need this to include exercise."

"Instead of just telling me to go to the gym, can you offer to watch the kids and give me time to go to the gym and have a few extra minutes for the sauna?"

"Instead of telling me to go for a walk, can you help me figure out how to catch up on sleep?"

"I'd like to have one night a week where we all find our own leftovers for dinner to free me up for exercise."

"I know it's my responsibility to find time to exercise. If you could encourage me every day to make this a priority, it would make me smile."

"I love you, and it's important to me that you know my time spent exercising is not meant as an escape from you, but a gift to myself."

"It's time to finally get a dog."

The above are examples to get you thinking. Your solutions and suggestions will be as unique as you and your relationships.

THIS IS YOUR NEW LIFE PRACTICE: THANK THEM.

BREAKING BARRIERS

WEEK THREE

See your barriers objectively and make a breakthrough!

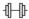

Exercise:

Go to Appendix C of this book and complete your exercise plans for Week 3.

Schedule your exercise plans into your calendar.

Lessons:

The Breaking Barriers List

Chillax

Walk

Want it Bad

Jiggle

THE BREAKING BARRIERS LIST

The Breaking Barriers List will change your life forever.

Today is the beginning of a two-week journey to break your barriers to exercise.

You will create a master list of the barriers that are holding you back from getting the exercise you need. Then you will spend time adjusting your attitudes toward the items in your list. As you work through the lessons, you will be able to see your barriers more objectively. You will get clarity on where to spend your energy breaking barriers and where to rest.

At the end of these two weeks, you will see your barriers to exercise in a whole new light and will be able to more effectively make breakthroughs with confidence.

Create Your Breaking Barriers List

The **Breaking Barriers List** tracks each and every barrier you have to exercise in your life. Nothing is off-limits. When you create your list, try not to censor yourself as you make your list. Also, just because something is a barrier to exercise doesn't mean you need to remove it from your life. You simply note it on your list.

Some of the items in your list will be barriers that will not change anytime soon. Below are a couple of hugely obvious examples of these types of barriers.

> *Lack of sleep caused by young children: Parents with infants rarely sleep through the night. A newborn infant causing sleep deprivation is definitely a barrier. While there might be adjustments parents can make to help their sleep, they still have an infant who will continue to wake them at night for months or years. This is a barrier to exercise that we would add to our list, even though it is obvious the baby is here to stay.*

> *A demanding full-time job: The job is not going away anytime soon, but we will still list this as a barrier to exercise.*

> *A hectic daytime routine: Parents with tween/teen kids spend a lot of time running around town, dropping kids off, chaperoning, sitting in the rain during soccer games, etc., plus making dinner, working, and running errands. The daytime routine is in constant flux with sport seasons and particular kid issues of the day. It's tough to set any routines.*

A major health issue: Health issues come and have the potential make us feel like we have failed, when in reality, we are simply experiencing a very normal part of being human. We will still list these as barriers to exercise.

....

There are many types of barriers to add to your list. Your barriers may include:

The Obvious
- *I have a job, kids, relationship, commute, major health issues.*
- *I have a 14-hour flight today.*

The Daily Grind
- *Tuesday's schedule is always over-packed.*
- *I just want a glass of wine when I get home.*
- *I'm already overwhelmed.*
- *I'm always exhausted.*
- *I accidentally brought two right-foot shoes to the gym, argh.*
- *The dog ate a pile of LEGO bricks, and now I'm headed to the vet.*

The Hidden
- *Every time I think of exercise my mind says, "Ugh!"*
- *I have health issues that I'm not aware of.*
- *I feel fat and ugly.*
- *I'm not worthy.*

When I was earnestly researching what it takes to create an active lifestyle, my list of barriers to exercise felt truly insurmountable. My **Breaking Barriers List** was huge. I was recently a single mom of a two-year-old who was often sick. I had to be out the door in a suit by 7:15 a.m. five days a week with my two-year-old and our lunches. My corporate clients were demanding. I rarely even mentioned I had a child, let alone that I was a single mother, because of the fear that people would see me as incapable. I remember one morning, my son threw up on the carpet in his room just before I needed to head out to an important client meeting. What did I do? I had no time, so I left the barf-carpet and headed to work. Carpet cleanup would have to wait until the evening. Long commutes meant even longer days with the added stress of picking up my child from daycare before it closed. By Friday, the house was always a disaster, and the weekends were spent playing catchup.

I hadn't yet learned how to set appropriate boundaries and to advocate for my space and time. I was everyone else's servant. I remember once actually crying when I finally made it to the gym—only to realize I had brought two right-footed tennis shoes! Overwhelmed, yes. Barriers to exercise? Absolutely. But I was highly-capable and proud of what I was able to accomplish despite my barriers.

We all have unique and amazing stories that shape how we are able to spend our days. Your story and list of barriers will be different from mine.

There are no wrong answers when you make your barriers list. If you see something in your life as a barrier to exercise, you are correct.

The takeaway for this lesson:
The only mistake you can make is to not dig deep enough. This is why you'll spend an entire week working though this, and then a second week making your breakthrough.

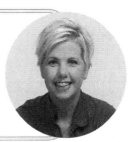

*I knew taking care of my kids full time took a lot of my time and energy, but I didn't realize just how much until I wrote out my **Breaking Barriers List**. Things like taking them to practice and coordinating schedules consumes my day. But the list also made me aware of the things that I could quickly and easily change. It pulled me out of making excuses and gave me a jump-start on owning my exercise. –Jason*

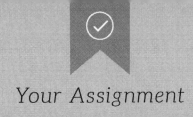

Your Assignment

PART ONE: *Create your Breaking Barriers List*

COLUMN 1: WHAT GETS IN MY WAY OF EXERCISING?

- List everything you can think of that gets in your way of exercising. Remember, there are no wrong answers. If it prevents you from exercising, write it down. Write down even the barriers that you already know are not going change. Everything counts.

COLUMN 2: WHAT ARE POSSIBLE SOLUTIONS FOR THIS ISSUE?

- In this column, write the first solution that comes to mind for each item in your list, then get creative and brainstorm additional solutions. It's okay to leave some of the solutions blank for now. Some of your items in the list are not going to change. This is all good.

Don't over-analyze anything; right now, you're just looking at data. You are working through making your barriers crystal clear to you. The more clarity you have on your barriers, the more power you will have to conquer the easy barriers, challenge the more difficult barriers, and embrace the barriers that are here to stay.

BREAKING BARRIERS

WHAT GETS IN MY WAY OF EXERCISING?	WHAT ARE POSSIBLE SOLUTIONS?
My job	Workout once a week at work.
My kids	Play/exercise with my kids each Saturday.
I have no energy	Look at my nutrition. Find a friend to get me going.
I hate the gym	Get creative. Find other ways to exercise.

PART TWO: Add to your list all week

Keep this **Breaking Barriers List** handy all week and add to it as more barriers come to mind. The more you think about it, the faster the ideas will come. You'll start to become more aware of those barriers, which inevitably brings attention to even more barriers. This is going to be a long list.

Use the notes pages in the back of this book to create your list.

BREAKING BARRIERS

WHAT GETS IN MY WAY OF EXERCISING?	WHAT ARE POSSIBLE SOLUTIONS?

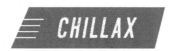

Before starting this lesson, take a moment and review your **Breaking Barriers List** from the previous lesson. Do you have anything else you can add to your list?

There's a good chance you have already started to break some of the barriers on your list. There's also a good chance that many of your barriers are items that aren't barriers at all, but rather restrictions you have placed on yourself.

HOW LONG IS YOUR LIST?

More realistically, your list is still mostly in your head, and you haven't taken the time to write it down yet. Yep—busted!

If this is you, take a couple more days to work on your **Breaking Barriers List** and then come back to this lesson.

READY TO ROLL NOW?

"How can I possibly relax when I have a mountain of barriers to face?!?"

Today, you are going to look at your **Breaking Barriers List** and complete one task that will help get you into a successful frame of mind.

Your task: Chillax.

Give yourself permission to relax while you face your full list of barriers to exercise. As you relax, continue to take an even closer look at the list you have created.

Relax and know that none of us will be solving our entire list today. Many barriers will stay right where they started: as barriers. This is perfectly fine. We don't need to break ALL of our barriers in order to make great progress. In fact, most of the items in your **Breaking Barriers List** will probably never shift. Don't let this discourage you. Instead, relax and know that reaching your goal doesn't require you to fashion a perfect life. Not at all. You will reach your goal despite the barriers that remain.

I have always had a life riddled with all kinds of barriers to exercise. If I wasn't dealing with an impossibly demanding job or the added load of being a single parent, then I was dealing with mysterious health issues stealing away my lung capacity. Never once has my life been in a place where I could say that even half of my barriers to exercise were resolved. However, the good news is that I never had to solve all of my barriers in order to make a breakthrough. I only had to solve just barely enough barriers to make a meaningful shift. Once I got to the point of making just enough breakthroughs, that's where magic happened, and I began to feel like my list was not so stifling.

I'm going to help you get to the space where you, too, have made the breakthroughs needed to live your active lifestyle. We have many lessons that are going to walk you through how to break free and live a life you love. However, before we start the hard work, I need you to first find a space where you can relax and give yourself compassion for the huge list of barriers in front of you. This is important.

Why This Is Important to You: Relaxing will give you energy.

The hero of any good story doesn't go around telling everyone how ridiculous their barriers are or how big the challenge is. They don't sit around in overwhelm and file complaints. Okay, maybe they do at first, but any good hero eventually manages to shake it off and take action. Good heroes get laser-focused on what they can do to conquer their barriers. If you find yourself getting uptight about issues in your life, it puts a strangle-hold on your ability to be strong. You'll get stuck in your issues and lose your ability to focus on solutions. You need to be your own hero.

When you take a moment to relax, pause, and breathe, you'll regain your center of balance and renew your energy. You'll have a better chance at maintaining focus on what is important, and you'll strike right at the heart of most issues. And you'll be in a better frame of mind to enjoy your life in the moment while at the same time creating a future you will love even more.

It's this positive energy that will carry you through the process.

RELAX. YOU'RE ALREADY ON YOUR WAY.

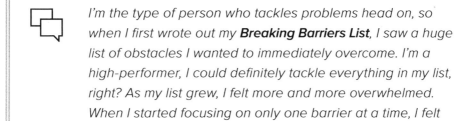

I'm the type of person who tackles problems head on, so when I first wrote out my **Breaking Barriers List***, I saw a huge list of obstacles I wanted to immediately overcome. I'm a high-performer, I could definitely tackle everything in my list, right? As my list grew, I felt more and more overwhelmed. When I started focusing on only one barrier at a time, I felt more in control and began to make real progress.* **–Zoe**

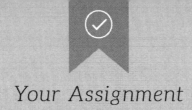

Your Assignment

PART ONE: *Relax*

Review your **Breaking Barriers List**. As you read through each item, practice relaxing around every issue that comes up for you. Notice the items in your list that cause you stress. Pause at each one and take a deep breath. Remind yourself that you do not need to solve it all today.

1. Read one item on your list.

2. Pause, relax, and breathe.

3. Repeat for all items in your list.

If you've never done an exercise like this before, it might feel a little strange or "woo-woo" to you. I can respect that. Remember, right now, it's just you sitting in a chair with this book. You are in full control of your mind; use it right now to find a sense of peace with your **Breaking Barriers List**.

PART TWO: *Reflections*

1. Take each of these statements below and very slowly repeat them several times.

I am making progress.
I am committed.
I am becoming a happier person.
I am finding joy.
I am worthy.

2. Pick ONE of the statements above and write it in large letters here.

3. Pause and look at the statement you wrote above. Why did this statement stand out to you? How it is relevant to your life today?

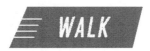

Are you wondering what walking could have to do with your Breaking Barriers List?

GREAT QUESTION!

In 2016, I transformed my life through walking. I made a big personal goal to walk 2,016 miles in the year 2016. Yes, that's a lot—about 5.5 miles a day. I actually wasn't sure if I would be able to complete the goal, especially since I had committed to completing all miles injury-free.

Originally, this goal was an ambitious way to keep me motivated and off the couch. I knew that if I went public with the goal, I'd be much more likely to succeed, because although I don't like to admit it, my ego can still highly motivate me. The goal was originally meant as simply a means to exercise consistently. I didn't know at the time that walking would literally change the trajectory of my life.

It gave me strong legs.
I connected with friends on a deeper level.
It gave my mind room to breathe.
It's where my best ideas showed up.
It gave me a daily boost of energy.

WALKING WAS SURPRISINGLY PRODUCTIVE TIME.

It didn't matter if I was walking in the rain, wind, mud, or darkness. Whether I was drinking water or sipping wine (that's right, late night slow strolls, I'll own it), walking gave me a break from the crazy and always returned me home ready to dance with life's curveballs again. Walking has been so profoundly good for my attitude and outlook on life that I've even given my husband permission to strongly encourage me to go for a walk when he sees I would benefit from some fresh air (aka: time for Mom to chill out).

The biggest and most unexpected piece was how walking changed the trajectory of my life. It was during those walks that the vision of COUCH to ACTIVE came to me. It was during those walks that I had my biggest revelations around how important it was for me to share what I had learned.

WOW.

Now it's your turn—begin to create YOUR walking story!

Walking is one of the most valuable exercises a human can do, yet it is all too often forgotten or dismissed. Walking will bring more value to your life than simply the walk itself; it will bring you peace of mind, clarity of thought, and a center and balance that you didn't have before.

In your upcoming assignment, we are going to use walking as a tool to help you clear your mind and give you the headspace to process your **Breaking Barriers List**. I can't look into a magic crystal ball and tell you what your mind will come up with; this will be your unique discovery.

Let's revisit your **Breaking Barrier List** in the assignment for this lesson.

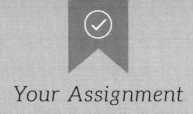

Your Assignment

PART ONE: *Plan your walk*

For the remainder of your COUCH to ACTIVE program, schedule a minimum of one solo walk a week.

1. Take a look at your calendar and schedule the best time for you to do a weekly solo walk.

2. Write your day and time in your calendar.

PART TWO: *Do the walk*

Before each of your solo walks, review your **Breaking Barriers List**. While you are on your walk, start by relaxing your mind. Here's how:

1. Lift your eyes up and look around. See everything that is interesting, beautiful, and curious.

2. Let your mind wander to how amazing it is that we are alive on this planet.

3. Breathe and remind yourself you are worthy of living a life you love.

4. Pause and don't worry about your **Breaking Barriers List**. Simply enjoy the walk.

Because you reviewed your **Breaking Barriers List** before your walk, your brain will already be working through solutions for you. The walk is going to help put your mind in a space where it can find solutions that are positive and create the life you desire.

You are relaxing.
You are breathing.
You are quite literally walking into a better space.

There is no written assignment for Part Two. Your assignment is to practice using walks as a way to clear your mind and breathe.

And yes, this is another life practice for you: go for a walk to clear your mind.

"WHAT IF I CAN'T WALK?"

Great question. If for any reason you are not able to walk, you can still do this exercise.

If you are unable to walk, then find about 20 minutes of quite time where you can relax and let your mind breathe. If you are able to be near nature, even better!

PART THREE: *Reflection*

When you return from your walk, complete these questions.

1. How did you feel at the end of your walk today?

2. How can you add more walking to your routine?

3. Do you need to make an investment in walking gear, such as a rain coat or winter clothes, to enable your walks?

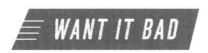

WANT IT BAD

Is this you? "I'm so frustrated with how impossible it is to exercise consistently." If you relate, that's fantastic! That's right, massive frustration around this topic is a good thing. When you are frustrated, it means you haven't given up. Your frustration ensures that the topic of exercise is still on your mind.

What if that is not you at all? What if you have been given this book as required reading? Or maybe your partner gave it to you, and you're working through the lessons because your partner asked you to? I hear you—this is a harder place to start from. You don't have the same internal motivation and are feeling a bit "meh" about the whole thing. The fact that someone else is having you read this is likely causing you to polarize in the opposite direction. You're going to need to rise above the fact that this book wasn't your idea and then still own your success. This is a big job, and I respect that.

Being frustrated enough to want the change in our life gives us energy to make a change.

THIS IS GOOD.

Wanting it badly fuels your fire to break barriers. It gives you the passion needed to stick with it. Being in touch with why this change is important to your unique life helps tremendously.

Amy is raising teenagers. I appreciate how in touch with reality her story is. Her reasons for change are unique to her. Let's take a look.

> "Although my recovery from the surgery was quick, my recovery from being sedentary wasn't, and I never really got back on track to maintain my weight loss.
>
> "Ten years is a blink, and before I knew it, I could no longer use the 'babies and toddlers' excuse for my weight. My kids were all teens and tweens, and the only person I had to blame for regaining those 35 pounds (plus about 20 more) was me. I was in my late 40s, exhausted, overweight, depressed, anxious, struggling to recover from the worst year of my life due to family struggles, lacking the basic confidence to do any of my old activities, and wondering if I had another 40 years to look forward to feeling the same way. I come from a long line of long-lived people; could I manage another 40 or more years of this?
>
> "And somewhere, a very deeply buried seed said, 'no.'

"No, I cannot go on like this. No, I will not live this way anymore. I am not weak. I am not worthless. I am more than a fat, lazy mom. No, these labels will not define me.

"It was a very quiet 'no' at first. On that 'no,' I found the strength to download a meal-tracking app. That 'no' pushed me to print a 12-week exercise plan and post it on the fridge. The 'no' got louder the first time I finished a full week of workouts, the first time I knitted instead of snacking, the first time I jogged 23 minutes without stopping....

"Before I knew it, I'd finished the first 12-week plan and printed another one. And then I did it again. And again. And the milestones kept coming, and I kept meeting them, and I kept going, all the while looking at the next milestone.

"It was not easy. There were a lot of voices trying to drown that 'no.' Some days, there was a veritable Mormon Tabernacle Choir in my head—'You're too busy today. Your kids need you more than you need the exercise. You need to be available. It's what good moms do—we sacrifice ourselves for our families. Don't you want to be a good mom? You're selfish for exercising. Besides, what good does it do? You'll just gain all the weight back eventually. You're almost 48—you don't need to look hot for anyone. This is futile. Just go eat potato chips.'

"I outran the voices."

....

Amy's "want it bad" came by polarizing against where she was in her life. She decided that she no longer wanted to feel exhausted, overweight, depressed, and anxious. It was enough for her to get the ball rolling. Since writing the story above, Amy has reached her goal weight and maintained her active lifestyle. Just last week she completed a multi-day backpack trip with her teenagers!

Wanting a change badly is great in theory. Now, let's take this concept and use a tool to harness the power of frustration to your advantage. We are going to get you to a space where you will no longer be spinning your wheels in aimless frustration.

If you are still feeling "meh" about putting in the work to create a change in your life, the assignment here will help you make the shift into action.

Your Assignment

In this assignment, we are going to take our frustration and use it to our greatest advantage. We are not going to completely alleviate all frustration you may be experiencing, and we are not going to solve every single item you may be frustrated about in your **Breaking Barriers List**. Instead, we are going to be strategic and focus on the most impactful progress requiring the least energy. You'll get clarity on where to focus your energy and gain confidence that you are using your frustration to your advantage so you can create a solution for your life.

Take another look at your **Breaking Barriers List**.

PART ONE: *Choose three items*

What are the top three items in your **Breaking Barriers List** that you're most passionate about? These could be the items that cause you the most stress or the ones you are most motivated to start solving for today. List those three items here.

Barrier #1 _____

Barrier #2 _____

Barrier #3 _____

PART TWO: *Dive deeper*

Now, take a closer look at each of these three barriers to exercise.

Barrier #1 _____

1. On a scale of 1-10, how badly do you want to change this barrier?

2. Is this something you can change today?

3. Is this something you can change in the future?

4. Do you want this to change? If yes, what action will you take now to get you closer to breaking this barrier?

Barrier #2 _____

1. On a scale of 1-10, how badly do you want to change this barrier?

2. Is this something you can change today?

3. Is this something you can change in the future?

4. Do you want this to change? If yes, what action will you take now to get you closer to breaking this barrier?

Barrier #3 _____

1. On a scale of 1-10, how badly do you want to change this barrier?

2. Is this something you can change today?

3. Is this something you can change in the future?

4. Do you want this to change? If yes, what action will you take now to get you closer to breaking this barrier?

There are probably items in your list that you are not going to be able to completely change today. This is perfectly fine. For now, focus on what you can do.

We have upcoming lessons that address what to do with barriers that are here to stay.

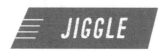

I'm going to take a subject that is painful for many of us and flip it on its head. I'm talking about the subject of body-image and the massive social pressure we put on ourselves to live up to completely unreal standards. In an effort to make things better, a massive wave of body-positive messaging has surfaced in mainstream media. The intentions around body-positive thinking are good, and I applaud the slow shift our culture is making in that direction.

However, there is still a critical gap between having the desire to love your body for what it is today and being able to love it in a way that feels genuine. I'm beginning to believe it's impossible. I hope I am wrong.

Before I jump into our topic of body image, here's why this topic is so critically important.

First of all, this is not just a women's issue. It's a human issue. It doesn't matter what gender you are. The topic of body image has come to a head in our culture. We already know that media constantly feeds us airbrushed images of perfection that don't exist in reality.

THIS IS JUST THE BEGINNING OF THE PROBLEM.

We are also bombarded daily with advertisements that deliberately prey on our insecurities in order to gain corporate profits. Most advertisements are designed to leave us feeling like we are lacking and need their magic gadget, program, powder, pill, or potion to make us feel happy, powerful, or cool. Back when I was primarily working with Fortune 500 companies, I sat in many boardroom meetings and received briefings from executives with Ph.D. degrees whose primary role for the company was to figure out how to manipulate people into clicking on ads and making a purchase. Much of this manipulation is aimed at making you feel like you have a gap in your life, you are flawed, or you are lacking in some way. I know this is standard procedure for most corporations with a product to sell. Regardless, I was floored by how humans can prey on each other for profit. I couldn't leave that soul-sucking corporate role fast enough. My point here is that the odds are stacked against us, and we're playing an unfair game.

As a result, body image issues span the entire spectrum of our population. I have several friends who are body builders; these athletes have obtained the pinnacle of health and fitness, yet still are incredibly self-critical. I'm connected with many health coaches who also struggle with the plague of their own body image. I know group fitness instructors who are closet bingers and starve themselves to ensure they continue to look like their product. Each year I attend a one-week conference of over one hundred health and fitness bloggers. As bloggers, you can imagine our online forums are very lively. Do you know what the number one hot-topic issue is for this group? You guessed it—body image. I've even known incredibly handsome and beautiful elderly people who are still self-critical of how their body looks. Body image issues are everywhere.

Even I struggle with body image at times. You read that right, your Bad Couch Guru was raised with the generation of Barbie® dolls, Aqua Net® extra super hold hairspray, and hot-pink legwarmers! I've had seasons in my life where I've been in wicked great shape and seasons of being very ashamed of gaining a few pounds of body fat. Ridiculous, I know! To make matters worse, I can be self-critical over how self-critical I am being.

When I reached my 40s, everything flipped on its head, and I came back for another round of revisiting body image in my own life. I know in my head that aging is normal and a perfect body doesn't matter. But matters of the heart are not as easy to settle. So I press on and defiantly refuse to let any bouts of body image issues restrict me from living a life I love. I choose to thrive!

With all of that said, here is my unique perspective on body image and the attitude we need to take toward how we see our own bodies, and how we show up in the world.

JIGGLE.

You're taking your amazing body out into the world and exercising.
You're going to jiggle.
That's right, I said it. Your thighs, waist, the triceps you've been hiding under those long sleeves for decades, are all going to jiggle. In other words, never let a body-image issue hold you back from living a life you love.

OWN IT AND CRACK A SMILE.

Now, I'm not asking anyone to belly dance on a street corner or go jogging in just a sports bra. Golly gee no! Especially you men—I'm not asking you to swim in a Speedo®. But if you insisted, and if you double-dog-dared me, I just might join you.

Negative body image issues are real. The hurt is real. The embarrassment is real. But you, my dear, are more wonderful than you realize. In fact, if you are still concerned about what others think, remind yourself that confidence is incredibly attractive. You can and you will work through this one.

The goal for this lesson is not to magically flip a switch and instantly love your body. Such a goal would be unrealistic, and I want you to feel the freedom in knowing that nothing is wrong with you in this struggle. Body image is a big topic that isn't resolved with a snap of the fingers.

Here's what you can do.

BE BRAVE.

Today, let's all take our jiggle and own it with pride. Let's be first in line to encourage each other for our bravery. Let's punch through our walls. You don't have to fully love your body before you can get out and live your life. Be the brave light who leads this dance. The world needs you to pave the path for others to see that yes, you can get out and jiggle and you won't die. In fact, you will thrive and we will love you for it. You will find allies. There are more people who will encourage you than discourage you. Let's find ourselves on the other side of this wall, standing in the sun in victory over our jiggly baggage.

Defiantly refuse to let any bouts of body image issues keep you from living a life you love!

Let's go jiggle!

 I spent too many years of my life feeling embarrassed of my body. I hid behind loose clothes and dreaded the summer months when it was too uncomfortably hot to wear long pants and sweaters. When I decided to adopt a body-positive attitude, things really changed for me. I decided I was tired of hiding, and I started figuring out how to love myself as I am. It's such a huge relief! I'm beginning to accept myself and believe that my self-worth is not tied to the shape of my body. Here's an interesting pro-tip: I don't have to fully love my body to get outside. In fact, getting outside as I am helps me conquer my fears. Nothing will stop me! —Zoe

Your Assignment

It is easy to tell others that they should get out there and exercise and not worry about whether or not they have a jiggly body, a bit of muffin top, or a lot of extra rolls around the waist.

But can you lead by example?

Now don't worry, I'm not going to ask you to put on a bikini or Speedo® and jump off the high dive. But I do want you to take a moment to pause and honestly assess whether or not your own body image issues are holding you back.

YOUR ASSIGNMENT IS TO MEMORIZE ONE OF THESE.

On the following page is a list of body-positive affirmations.

1. Pick the one affirmation on the following page that speaks to you the most clearly and honestly.

2. After this list of affirmations is an entire page dedicated to the affirmation you select. Write this ONE affirmation in big letters on that page.

3. Memorize it.

4. **Bonus:** Write it on a sticky note and place it somewhere you will see it.

BODY-POSITIVE AFFIRMATIONS

My body loves me, and I will love it back.

I am strong, I am beautiful, I am enough.

I do not value my body over my being.

My goal is to fall in love with everything I am.

My body, my shape, my rules.

This is what progress looks like.

Being sexy is all about attitude, not body type.

Life is way too short to spend another day at war with myself.

I'm not going to sacrifice my mental health to have the perfect body.

I'm obsessed with becoming a person comfortable in my own skin.

I said to my body, "I want to be your friend." It took a long breath and replied,
"I have been waiting my whole life to hear this."

I exercise because I love my body, not because I hate it.

My body is not an ornament; it's a vehicle to my dreams.

My body is a gift, and I embrace my body with love and respect.

It's time for me to unlearn everything society has taught me about hating
my body.

My self-worth is not determined by a number on the scale.

My imperfections make me beautiful.

When I fuel my body with love, my mind has no limits.

I am not a mistake or a problem to be solved. I am limitless.

I love and accept all parts of myself.

I am grateful for my body and don't compare myself to others.

I am putting my life in order and preparing to accept all the good that is coming to me.

I do not have to like everything about myself in order to love myself.

I am attracting powerful, positive, and healthy people into my life.

I am proud of how far I have come and have faith in how far I will go.

MY AFFIRMATION

Write your affirmation here in big bold letters.

The takeaway for this lesson:
Be the brave light who leads this dance.
You will not just survive, you will thrive.
We will love you for it.

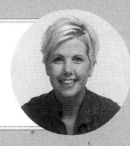

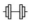

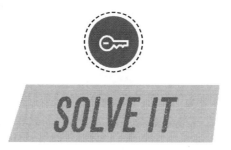

WEEK FOUR

Strategies to break barriers and create a life you love!

Exercise:

Go to Appendix C of this book and complete your exercise plans for Week 4.

Schedule your exercise plans into your calendar.

Lessons:

Barrier Zones

Naysayers

Mini-Solutions

Jump

Try it All

Impossible to Flake

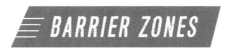

BARRIER ZONES

I'm going to guide you through a process of prioritizing your barriers list. This exercise will pull you out of overwhelm and land you in a space where you are completely objective about what is getting in your way. You will no longer be able to be apathetic or sluggish or use excuses. You will own where you are and what you are going to do about it.

Breaking down your long list into different types of barriers will help you create a plan of attack, which gives you more control over them. Some of your barriers are outside of our control, some are temporary, and some are here to stay. You are going to classify your barriers into these categories, and then work through each category one at a time.

Temporary vs. Permanent Barriers

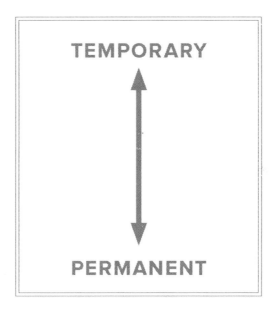

For the purpose of this lesson, a permanent barrier is an item on your list that will not change for at least one year. Your body sees a full year of a routine as permanent; it doesn't know that you are in the middle of a high-pressure career or that retirement is only a few years away. All your body knows is that right now, you are not exercising.

Temporary barriers are all of things that get in your way, but are either a one-time event or will soon change. These are typically little things like a project at work, the daily grind of managing kids, getting stuck in a traffic jam, and general adult responsibilities. These also include the speed bumps of life such as illness, injury, and caring for our aging loved ones.

Out of My Control vs. I Can Influence

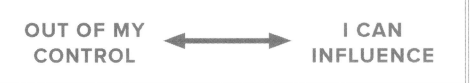

OUT OF MY CONTROL ⟷ I CAN INFLUENCE

It's time for you to get resourceful and objective about what barriers you can influence vs. what barriers are truly out of your control. How much can you really do to affect them? How much relies on external forces like the people around you, your job, or the environment that surrounds you? Many barriers have both an element that we can influence and a piece that is out of our control.

The key lies in identifying which elements of each barrier can make a positive shift. Overall, the barrier might stay intact, but there are definitely small adjustments you can make within the barrier that will make a big difference.

THE KEY TO CHANGE BEGINS WITH AWARENESS.

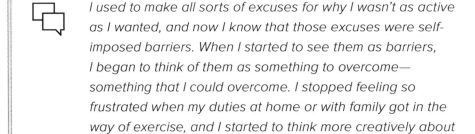

I used to make all sorts of excuses for why I wasn't as active as I wanted, and now I know that those excuses were self-imposed barriers. When I started to see them as barriers, I began to think of them as something to overcome— something that I could overcome. I stopped feeling so frustrated when my duties at home or with family got in the way of exercise, and I started to think more creatively about the ways that I could overcome those barriers. That mindset shift was a game changer for me. −Jason

Here are a few examples:

Parents with young children can't control when their children wake at night. However, they can be conscious about putting down electronic devices and sleeping when they have the opportunity.

. . . .

Acute illness can prevent us from exercising. We generally can't control the illness. However, we can be more intentional about eating right and staying hydrated to help prevent illness, and we can control how we care for our bodies to encourage a quick recovery.

. . . .

An aging parent who needs care can limit our time to exercise. However, many times our aging parents are happy when we lovingly tell them we need to exercise. It helps them to feel like less of a burden when they see us caring for ourselves.

. . . .

If we are on a high-pressure project at work, getting away to exercise can seem all but impossible. However, when you remember that we are all humans and we all need time to exercise, you are more empowered to help lead the team with healthy habits.

. . . .

Annoying things like getting a parking ticket or a bad haircut can wreck our afternoon. But if we identify these upfront as mere annoyances, we don't have to let them wreck our plans for the rest of the day.

. . . .

Our ability to influence our barriers will vary from day to day, which is perfectly fine. When we can spot the difference between what we can and cannot influence, it becomes even easier to manage it all. The key to making changes and breaking down barriers begins with awareness. Once you're aware of the barriers in front of you, you can begin to break them down in a methodical way.

All barriers fit somewhere within the matrix below. Each barrier has elements of permanent and temporary and factors you can influence and control. Each also has elements completely outside of your control.

Let's break down the matrix a bit further.

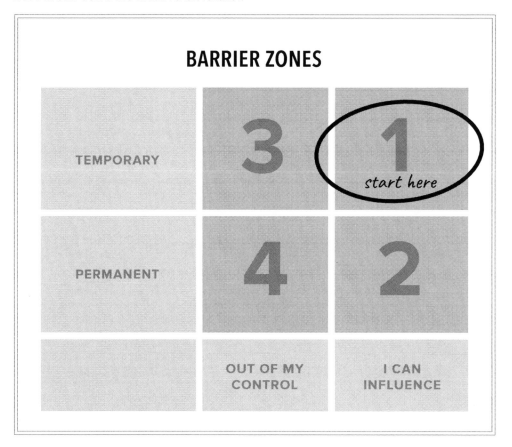

ZONE 1: Temporary Barriers I Can Influence

Start with these first. They are the easiest, in-the-moment barriers you can break daily. Picture yourself as a ninja breaking through these barriers. One barrier at time, you are finally taking control of your life and shifting it in the direction you've always wanted it to go. These quick successes will bring you energy, and you'll quickly see positive changes in your life.

ZONE 2: Permanent Barriers I Can Influence

These barriers are in your life for more than one year, but you can influence them. These are the items on your list that are definitely solvable, but not overnight. Working toward solutions with these barriers brings a huge sense of fulfillment to your life!

ZONES 3 & 4: Barriers Out of My Control

At times, you'll face challenges or phases of life that are here to stay, at least for the foreseeable future. When you identify these situations, work through the following process to keep your progress healthy.

Steps to take when a barrier is here to stay:

1. Challenge yourself: Is this really a Zone 3 or Zone 4 Barrier? Or am I in some way limiting myself?

2. Respect the fact that this is not going to change today.

3. Give yourself compassion.

4. If this is a lifetime permanent barrier, resolve to come to peace with your unique situation.

5. There are times in our lives when we decide that a situation we previously viewed to be permanent and out of our control (Zone 4) is actually something we can change with massive action on our parts (Zone 2).

We will address permanent barriers in more detail during week six of this book.

Why This Is Important to You: You can influence the barriers to your health.

When you realize that you don't need to solve every barrier, you are in a better space to focus on the barriers you can impact.

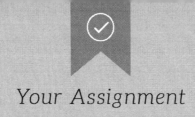

Your Assignment

In this assignment, you are going to look through your **Breaking Barriers List** and gain more clarity on what types of barriers you are facing.

PART ONE: *Assign a Number*

1. Go back to your **Breaking Barriers List** and review each item.

2. Assign a barrier zone level to every item in the list. Write the zone level next to each item.

PART TWO: *Pick Two*

1. Look at your barriers list and circle ONE Zone 1 item that you will conquer TODAY. Pick the item that looks like the easiest item to conquer. What item did you select? Write it here.

2. Circle ONE Zone 2 barrier you will begin to work on TODAY. Again, pick the easiest item you labeled Zone 2. What item did you select? Write it here.

3. Sometime TODAY, break through the two barriers you selected.

NOTE ABOUT THIS ASSIGNMENT: Most of us will want to start conquering as many items in the list as possible right away. For today, resist the temptation and instead focus on just the two easier items you circled. After you have conquered these two, then you can revisit more items in your list.

This is your new life practice. You are objectively seeing your barriers and effectively working your fastest route to success. This internal work is hugely important, and it's something that separates people who successfully transition to an active lifestyle from those who don't.

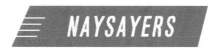
NAYSAYERS

Not everyone is going to jump on board and be supportive. Some will be downright negative. Naysayers come in all shapes and sizes. It could be a coworker who makes passive-aggressive comments about your health choices or a loved one who reminds you over and over of failed attempts in the past. Heck, it could even be a complete stranger or even your own negative self-talk subconsciously sabotaging your efforts.

Even the most wonderful and amazing people can say the dumbest things. When you experience this, remember you are not alone. Every single one of us on this journey will encounter naysayers, people who don't believe in us, and others who think they know us better than we know ourselves.

When you encounter negative, hurtful, or ignorant statements, here's what you do:

IGNORE THEM.

Don't give them your attention. Instead, use these statements to fuel your determination to meet your goal.

Stay the course and focus on the amazing work you are doing. Remind yourself of the awesome new life you are creating—

POSITIVE, EMPOWERED, AND STRONG.

Focus on the friends who encourage you. If you don't have anyone encouraging you today, don't fear. You will find them. They are there.

I've had a tremendous amount of naysayers in my life. Some were more toxic than others. I've had a doctor tell me that a 15-minute workout is as good as worthless. He was wrong. I had a mean friend who said I looked like a duck when I ran. He was right, but I still let it hurt me back then. I had a friend ask me, "What are you trying to prove?" Ignoring their stabs was always the right move.

Naysayers can also be complete strangers. Below is a story Anne shared that struck right to my heart and made me want to chase down this naysayer and give her a piece of my mind. Anne was in the middle of an amazing life transformation. She had lost 70 pounds in eight months by eating right and working out hours every day. Anne was still actively working to lose another 50 pounds when she shared this story.

"When you're overweight you have to carry around a lot more than excess pounds. Sometimes it's roiling indignant anger, even 24 hours after the fact. When one of your neighbors tells you to take the stairs instead of the elevator 'because a little exercise every once in a while wouldn't hurt you' it takes a phenomenal amount of self-control not to respond in kind. I don't think I'm mad at her anymore, not really, but mad at myself for allowing her to hurt me. I'm so proud of everything I've accomplished regarding self-image, but this incident made me realize that the work of realizing your own self-worth never ends. And it's an exhausting prospect."

It takes an incredible amount of strength to make a significant change in your life, even if that change is a positive one. It takes even more strength to continue to pursue your goals like Anne did despite having naysayers in her life. I applaud Anne for the progress she continues to make. She is an amazing human.

There are times when the naysayer in your life cannot be ignored. Let's take a look at Skylar who has an incredibly loving partner who just doesn't get it.

"My partner loves me more than anything in the world, but when I started to exercise, he just didn't get it. He had never exercised since his college days. He would tell me daily that people who run get injured, so I shouldn't run. I started jogging secretly because I didn't want to hear his comments about runners and injury. We still loved each other very much, but I knew this dynamic between us was messed up. Still, I continued my silent defiance of exercising daily. One day while I was jogging, I fell and twisted my ankle badly. I panicked about the thought of calling him and getting the 'I told you so' lecture. I was in crutches for weeks. It was during this time in crutches that I came clean and told him I was jogging. What happened next shocked me. He cried and told me that the real reason he has been so negative about my exercise was because, deep down, he was afraid that if I got in amazing physical shape, I might leave him. Wow. I truly didn't see that coming! The healing between us was long overdue, and he never again put me down for exercising or jogging."

Wow. What would have happened to Skylar if they never had that critical conversation?

Why This Is Important to You: Naysayers drain your energy.

It's tempting to focus on negative influences headed your way. When someone puts you down, it's natural to get defensive and want to solve it. But in this case, it's important that you simply ignore it and move on. You will do better by focusing your energy on the positive work you are doing in your life. Don't get distracted by a naysayer.

Is it really this simple? For the most part, yes it is. You are becoming more and more empowered with your life and the direction you want your future to go. You now realize you are worthy of creating this in your life, and you are learning how to bring others into your circle in a positive way. So yes, you can ignore the naysayers. Have patience. Show them kindness and compassion. You don't need to explain yourself to a naysayer. Let the life you live be the example. Be patient, strong, and resilient. They will eventually see, and then they might even want to be more like you.

It takes a great deal of courage to ignore the naysayers, and it can be even harder if your naysayer is someone that you must deal with, but you can do it. You've already taken so many positive steps—this is just one more step on the path to your goals.

*When I started to be more active, I had a lot of trouble with one of my close friends. She would remind me about my wasted gym membership, the yoga program I never finished, and the time I told everyone I was going to do a marathon but instead ditched it for yet another massive work project. She even went out of her way to try to schedule a girls' weekend when she knew I was planning on finally doing a bubble run. I didn't understand why my friend would passive-aggressively sabotage me; she's smarter than that. After much reflection, I realized that she was afraid of losing me as a friend. She was afraid I wouldn't like her anymore. What?!? She's one of my best friends! I made a big effort to reassure her that she is my dear friend, no matter what. I didn't even need to address her negativity, and thankfully, she stopped being so negative. It was bizarre, but it worked. **–Zoe**

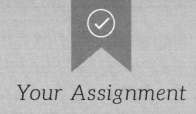

Your Assignment

There is no written assignment for this lesson. Instead, find a quiet space to work through these exercises.

PART ONE: *Imagine your naysayers*

I am going to guide you through an exercise where you will use your imagination to break through the negative influence naysayers have on you. Spend a little extra time really processing through this one.

IMAGINE THIS:

Pick one or two people in your life who have been your biggest naysayers. I want you to imagine their criticism or doubt of you. Imagine their critical words floating toward you, and just as those words approach you, step aside and let their hurtful words flow on by. Don't grab those critical words and throw them back. And don't stand there motionless letting the critical word strike your heart.

Instead, imagine having compassion for your naysayers. Imagine yourself standing tall and knowing you will succeed with or without their support. Your success is not dependent on their opinions.

Now imagine yourself one year from today. You succeeded. Your naysayers forgot they were ever critical, or, deep down, they are proud of the positive change you made for yourself. The struggle to defend against the naysayer is now a non-issue for you.

PART TWO: *Consider your value*

Do you have a big naysayer in your life? Right now, make the decision that the joy of your new active lifestyle is more valuable to you than the negative words. Decide that the naysayer's negative vibe doesn't deserve your energy. You are not going to let those words hold you down, no matter how relentless the naysaying may be. **You do not need permission to improve your life. You are worthy.**

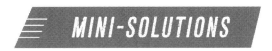

We are going to take the concept of "movement is movement" and unpack this further.

You don't need a perfect workout plan to be a person who exercises consistently. As long as you are juggling so many priorities, you need the freedom to be nimble and flexible with exercise.

YOUR SUCCESS IS NOT GOING TO FIT NEATLY INTO A BOX.

I love training for events and challenging myself to see what my body is capable of. I love doing this even though I have health issues that keep me far from any medal or podium finish. However, there have been seasons in my life where training for a specific event was unrealistic. Back when I was a single mom with a long commute, demanding clients, and a sick child, I also had a wave in my life where seven people in my family died, three quite tragically. It was during that time in my life that I would get angry when I'd hear platitudes like, "you have the same 24 hours in a day as everyone else," or even worse, "if it was important to you, you'd make it a priority." Those platitudes were not true for me. We don't always have the same 24 hours, and sometimes we do have competing priorities.

You heard me right: sometimes our priorities correctly steer us away from realistically being able to commit to rigid exercise plans. The good news is that we can get in the exercise we need without a rigid exercise plan. If you use this strategy to the max, you can pretty much get the exercise your body needs. Now, it's no secret that to train for a specific event, you must follow a specific plan. We'll address that more in a few minutes.

For these seasons in our lives when it truly seems too crazy to be able to commit to the time you think you need, mini-solutions are one of the most powerful tools we can use to keep movement and exercise going despite the crazy-as-bananas circumstances we are actively working through.

I call this the "mini-solution" approach.

MINI-SOLUTIONS ARE POWERFUL.

These are all of the small things you can do throughout your day and year that add up to an active lifestyle.

Your mini-solutions are designed to change the way you look at exercise. They will help you get exercise you wouldn't normally fit in by not compartmentalizing exercise to only the times you are "officially" exercising.

Mini-solutions we already know:

- *Take the stairs instead of the elevator.*

- *Park farther from your destination.*

- *Go for a walk during your lunch break.*

We know these already, and many of us are probably already doing some of these. Mini-solutions can range from something you do at the spur of the moment to an event you do once a year. The best mini-solutions fit these criteria:

- *They help you get exercise you might not get otherwise.*

- *They help you make exercise happen on days that feel too busy.*

- *They make you smile.*

Below are examples of other mini-solutions:

- *Your kids are at a playground; how can you join in? Let your childlike nature come alive.*

- *The Parks and Recreation catalogue arrives, and you feel adventurous. Do something new!*

- *Your gym has classes you've never tried. It's time to be brave.*

- *You've always wanted to build that rock wall in the back yard, haven't you?*

- *There's a dance class in town you've always been too shy to try—until now.*

- *How well do you really know your town? Start walking.*

- *It's pouring down rain, and you need some time alone. You have a raincoat and walking shoes, right?*

- *You're standing in line—100 calf raises!*

- *You spend a year inviting friends to exercise with you; now they are finally starting to invite you, too.*

- *You create a new holiday tradition that includes exercise.*

- *You look for vacation destinations that include exercise you enjoy.*

- *You make a conscious decision to not habitually turn on the TV.*

- *You find pieces of work clothes that can also function for not-so-sweaty exercise breaks.*

- *You update to a more carefree hairstyle.*

- *You keep a pair of tennis shoes in your car at all times.*

- *You re-arrange your living room furniture to make room for a yoga mat and a few weights.*

The more specific your mini-solutions are to your unique life, the better.

We get stuck when we try to fit into someone else's box. Mini-solutions give you ways to move more. Trust your gut. Go with what makes you smile.

Mini-solutions also tie in with your Breaking Barriers List. Here are a few examples:

Breaking Barriers List Item: I'm always so tired.
Mini-Solutions: I'll set a daily alarm for 10 pm on my phone to help remind me to go to sleep. I will allow myself to sleep all day this Saturday. On my next vacation, I'll plan in time to pack so that it's not a huge rush the night before I depart.

Breaking Barriers List Item: Cooking for the family takes so much time.
Mini-Solutions: I'll allow as many days a week as possible to be "leftovers day," and I will relax and let the family find their own dinner. I'll give myself permission to

order healthy takeout at least once a week. I'll intentionally plan a couple of meals with significantly less prep time. I'll give myself permission to join a meal-prep service.

Breaking Barriers List Item: My job sucks out every bit of energy I have.
Mini-Solutions: I'll keep a pair of tennis shoes at my desk and do a ten-minute walk when possible. I'll park as far away from the entrance as possible and take the stairs. I'll walk to the restroom that is farther away from my desk. I'll learn how to do stretches at my desk. If a standing desk is an option, I'll do that. I'll start seriously thinking about whether I need an attitude adjustment for my job or if I need an entirely new job.

Mini-solutions are a powerful tool that can get you to a place of success even if you don't have everything figured out right now. In fact, mini-solutions can help you succeed even if you NEVER feel like you've got it all under control.

MINI-SOLUTIONS ARE FOR EVERYONE.

You don't have to be going through a particularly crazy time in your life for mini-solutions to be meaningful. Anyone can layer on mini-solutions to the exercise they do. Whether you are training for your first 5K, working toward a bodybuilding competition, or want to up your performance in a team sport, layering on mini-solutions to your training will give you an added advantage.

My mother was dying from cancer at the same time I was juggling a massive project at work and parenting my own children. Sometimes just getting out of bed to deal with it all felt almost insurmountable. For that period in my life, something had to give. I made the difficult decision to pause my dance classes, and instead, I exercised whenever possible. Sometimes it was a 15-minute jog around my mom's neighborhood; other days it was as simple as walking up and down the ten-story stairwell at the office a few times a day. It was an incredibly tough season in my life, and I'm glad I'm not there anymore. But I am grateful I was able to use the concept of mini-solutions to patch me through. **–Zoe**

Your Assignment

PART ONE: *Mini-solutions for life*

Take a second look at the examples of mini-solutions in this lesson. Create your own list of mini-solutions that can help you keep exercising more. Whether you are just beginning to exercise or are training for an elite event, mini-solutions work for all of us.

MY MINI-SOLUTIONS

MINI-SOLUTIONS WORK

1. Pack tennis shoes in car.

2. List friends I will start inviting out for walks.

3. Play with kids when we are at the playground.

4.

5.

6.

7.

8.

9.

10.

11.

12.

13.

14.

PART TWO: *Discover mini-solutions in your Barriers List*

Open to your **Breaking Barriers List**. Read through your list again and look for any items that can be solved, or partially solved, through a mini-solution. Add any new items to your list above.

PART THREE: *Your life practice*

MEMORIZE THIS:

Mini-solutions work.

I will succeed even if I don't have it all figured out.

This is your new life practice: Mini-solutions work.

MINI-SOLUTIONS HELP YOU SUCCEED EVEN IF YOU NEVER FEEL LIKE YOU'VE GOT IT ALL UNDER CONTROL.

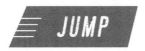

You've got to be on your toes for this step. It is easy to miss.

Every day we respond and react to everything around us. We sort through countless micro-decisions every day. Micro-decisions add up to our days, which add up to our weeks, months, years, and life. You get it.

Our real power is in each moment-to-moment opportunity that floats our way and then passes by.

WHEN AN OPPORTUNITY TO EXERCISE COMES YOUR WAY, JUMP ON IT!

Don't make excuses. Don't rationalize. Don't assume you can exercise later in the day. Don't say "that flight of stairs won't count for much."

DON'T LET OPPORTUNITIES FLOAT AWAY. JUMP!

Opportunities that float our way:

- *A flight of stairs instead of escalator. (Oh, you've heard that one before?)*

- *A friend who would love to exercise with you—if you asked.*

- *A garage that needs cleaning, a yard that needs weeding, etc.*

- *An exercise class that could change your life.*

This is especially important when you see an opportunity that looks like fun and will make you smile. Don't get stuck seeing yourself as serious mature adult. Tap into your playful, childlike side that sees the world as a playground. Give yourself the freedom to let loose and have some fun.

Decide now that you WILL jump when the opportunity comes. Don't let your brain trick you out of an opportunity to succeed. JUMP! (Now say "jump" ten times fast!)

Your Assignment

PART ONE: *Memorize this*

JUMP!

I jump on every opportunity to exercise.

I am resourceful.

Now, close your eyes and repeat the passage in your mind multiple times.

PART TWO: *Jump*

List areas in your life where you can jump on exercise.

1. _____

2. _____

3. _____

4. _____

This is your new life practice.

JUMP!

 Some of my son's friends decided that they wanted to go play laser tag. Normally I'd sit in the lobby and wait for them to finish. This time, I decided to jump in, and I asked a friend to meet me there so we could play, too. It was a blast! I connected with my son, got my exercise, and now—I can't wait to go back again! **–Jason**

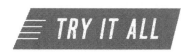

Hey you—super serious adult with a job and a mortgage and taxes to pay: are you in a rut?

As adults, it's easy to get into a rut. We don't mean to; it just happens. Trying all different kinds of exercise can be so powerful for our body and spirit. The adrenaline rush of trying something new is a great way to energize yourself and break out of a rut. You know this, but what holds you back from doing it?

Most of us forget that when we talk about exercise, we are referring to anything that gets our bodies moving:

- *Playing with our kids/grandchildren.*

- *Dancing in your kitchen when nobody's watching. (You can even dance when someone is watching!)*

- *Intentionally doing squats while picking up items.*

- *Getting up from your desk every hour and walking for five minutes.*

All of those types of exercise are valid. When you find something new that you love, something that makes you smile, you'll become truly energized.

Breaking Through Your Stereotypes

Are you limited by the stereotypes you have about who does what type of exercise? One key to breaking out of a rut and trying new things is breaking through stereotypes. Do you find yourself saying "I'm not a dancer" or "yoga's not for me"?

I want to encourage you to break out of your own stereotypes of where you think you will be accepted and fit in. Give something new a try. By trying something new, you are giving yourself a gift. You are not just expanding your exercise options; you're expanding your outlook on life.

Challenge yourself to clearly see the stereotypes you hold about different kinds of exercise:

- *Do you think water aerobics is just for the old, fat, or injured?*

- *Do you think ballet is only for the skinny girls?*

- *Do you think swing dancing is only for coordinated people?*

- *Do you wonder if yoga is only for those "woo-woo" people?*

- *Do you find yourself saying cycling classes are only for the hard-core people?*

I have either taught or tried pretty much every form of exercise. What has always stood out to me is the fact that the stereotypes of who does what kind of exercise are never entirely true for ANY of these. There are all kinds of people doing all kinds of activities. There are people already out there blazing this trail for you.

I have completed the Seattle to Portland 200-mile bicycle ride six times. Before I ever did this event, I had a very strong stereotype in my head that you had to be a lean and mean, super-fit, Tour de France type of athlete to complete 200 miles in two days. I wondered if I could one day do the event, but at the time thought it was completely out of my reach. There was one year where I had a few friends who were doing the event and needed someone to drive their support car. I spent two days watching the thousands of cyclists ride, stop for food, wait in long porta-potty lines, sleep in tents, and then do it all again for a second day. I was amazed at all of the different ages and body types. Virtually nobody fit my stereotype of a person who completed this type of ride. Grandparents, young teenagers, people with 100 pounds to lose were all enjoying the event. Even more striking was that everyone was so friendly and having a ripping great time! On day two, I spent hours at the finish line watching the cyclists arrive. I decided that I, too, would someday become a Seattle to Portland finisher!

My wife talks all the time about how much she loves her yoga classes and asks me to come along with her. But I always felt like I'd be uncomfortable there, surrounded by a bunch of flexible women. Finally, she talked me into taking a class, and I learned just how wrong I was. There were four other guys in the class, and the class was filled with people of all different ages and abilities. I totally had a stereotype in my head of people who go to yoga classes, and I was completely off-target. I actually really enjoyed myself! Seriously friends, give anything a try. What's the worst that could happen? **–Jason**

Why This Is Important to You: You are not a stereotype!
So many times, we hold ourselves back for no good reason. The people who are willing

> **JOIN THE TRAILBLAZERS. TRY IT ALL.**
> **TRY SOMETHING NEW, AND DEFY YOUR**
> **OWN STEREOTYPES OF WHAT YOU ARE CAPABLE**
> **OF OR WHAT YOU MIGHT ENJOY.**

to be brave and try something new come alive simply by trying something new.

The more options you see for yourself, the easier it is to be active.

Here are a few ideas to get you thinking:

- *If you have a gym membership, try every single group fitness class they offer. You can always start in the back of the room by the door to make an exit if it really is that bad.*

- *If you are working with a personal trainer, tell your trainer about your assignment to get creative and ask your trainer to try something new with you.*

- *Go to YouTube and search for exercise videos. Fair warning on these, though. Most YouTube fitness videos are difficult, and they will not accommodate your unique physical needs. Stay injury-free!*

- *Do something fun outdoors (hiking, biking, kayaking, swimming, beach walks).*

- *Join a community sport—kickball, volleyball, soccer, etc. There are many unique teams out there that focus primarily on having fun.*

- *Sign up for a wacky run/walk. There are all kinds of bubble runs, turkey trots, color dashes, and beer runs that are designed specifically for people who love to have fun while exercising.*

- *Try something completely different—ballroom dancing, karate, yoga, ballet, spring training camp, fencing, sword fighting, horseback riding, snorkeling, climbing.*

- *Try a great workout that is also gentle on the joints—chair yoga, Silver Sneakers, cycle class, aqua aerobics, Pilates, foam rolling.*

- *Go on a vacation that is centered around exercise. Google search "exercise vacations" or "fitness vacations," and you'll discover an endless list of opportunities.*

- *Volunteer anywhere that physical labor is needed.*

- *Help a friend organize his or her garage.*

STAY OPEN-MINDED AND THINK COMPLETELY OUT OF THE BOX.

Tips for Success:

- *Don't decide immediately if you like the activity; just ask yourself if you'd be willing to try it a few more times.*

- *Push your limits, but don't feel pressured by others to do anything you don't want to do.*

- *If you take a group exercise class, do empower yourself to modify as you need to in order to stay injury-free. There's nothing wrong with staying in the back of a group fitness class and doing what you can.*

- *Do tell your friends about your experience.*

When you stay open-minded, refuse to buy into stereotypes, and try new things, your life will come alive. This is true for all of life, isn't it?

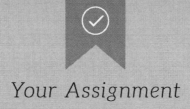

Your Assignment

PART ONE: *Try something new*

It's time to expand your horizons and try a new exercise or activity. Pick one exercise or exercise-related activity that you either haven't done in a long time or would like to try. Pick one even if you already feel like you know what types of exercises you like. The point is to expand your comfort zone and develop a willingness to try new ways to exercise.

1. What exercise did you pick?

2. Open your calendar and make a plan for when you are going to try the exercise or activity within the next month. Write your plan here.

TRY IT ON

EXERCISE	WHEN
Weekend dancing	Next Saturday night
Bubble Run	This July
Kayaking Lessons	This August
Chair Yoga	Tomorrow

PART TWO: *Make this a new life practice*

After you complete PART ONE above, continue trying new exercises as a life practice. Always keep your eyes open for new ways to exercise, new activities you can try, and new ways to expand your horizons. Never limit yourself or allow yourself to be put into a box. Have courage. You are limitless!

Create a list of other exercises you might like to try.

KEEP IT FRESH AND MAKE IT FUN.

Do this and you will create an active lifestyle you love.

TRY IT ON

EXERCISE	WHEN

IMPOSSIBLE TO FLAKE

If you base your entire exercise program on this lesson alone, you will end up in fantastic shape. But if you follow this lesson blindly and don't incorporate the mental shift here, it could leave you stressed out and miserable. So be smart and use this lesson to enhance your love of exercise, not destroy it. Ensure it makes sense for you.

REMEMBER, YOUR GOAL IS TO CREATE A LIFE YOU LOVE.

Make it Impossible to Flake

When you find yourself stuck in a space where you are so busy doing everything for everyone else that you can't make time to exercise, there are actions you can take to make it impossible to flake on your exercise plans. Add a level of accountability that creates a situation where you would never flake out on your exercise plans, even if other important distractions come your way. This looks different in everyone's life. You'll need to figure out how this will play out in your life.

"I'M NOT FLAKING OUT. NOT TODAY."

The most obvious example of this life practice is to join a team sport or get a small part-time job as a coach or instructor. This level of commitment will have a dramatic improvement on your chances of showing up for the exercise. You won't want to let the team or your employer down.

Here are a few examples of how this concept plays out.

> ***Rick joined a league:*** *"I'm an information technology specialist. I spend most of my time coding for a large software corporation you might have heard of before. I knew my company had a softball league, but didn't think much of it until my buddy at work told me they needed another player to fill out the team. I had never played before and wasn't sure if they would accept someone like me. Not only did they accept me, I fit right in. We are all software geeks. You can't help but laugh when teams Python and Java play to see who will come out on top. Aside from the bad programming joke, I appreciate how the company supports exercise in a way that is fun and makes it easy for me to show up."*

Mark and Susan lead a league: *Mark and Susan cherish their time together with each other and their teenagers. They are both busy professionals, and their priority right now is to spend more time with their kids. When their kids joined the local mountain biking chapter, they signed up as ride leaders. They were surprised by how supportive the chapter was in training them as leaders. Mark and Susan now get to spend more time with each other and their teenagers, and they are getting in the same big biking workouts as the teenagers are in their mountain biking chapter. Because they are leaders and the team depends on them, they never miss a ride. They're in great shape!*

When I was in high-demand senior management roles, I learned that it's pretty easy for someone like me to earn a group fitness certification. This gave me the ability to teach at my local gym. It was pretty great to get paid to work out rather than having to pay for a gym membership! Plus, I never miss any of my teaching workouts because I'm am the teacher—I have to be there!

In each of these examples, all of us are getting so much more done than just exercising. Rick is making connections with colleagues. Mark and Susan have a whole new active lifestyle that includes time with their teenagers. I have an outlet for my hugely extroverted personality.

Let's start thinking about how this could play out in your life.

Keep this in mind: While this form of forcing a workout is incredibly effective, it adds a layer of stress because you've put yourself in a position where it is impossible to flake. As a group fitness instructor, I've had a few bumps where the lack of flexibility frustrated me and made my life temporarily stressful. But overall, I absolutely love it, so it's worth it to me. Make sure the added stress is worth the joy of the activity you choose. There's no wrong or right answer here.

There's one more caveat we must add to help dial in the intention of this life practice. There may be a situation where you set up an exercise scenario that is impossible to flake on, but something unavoidable arises, and you still flake. For example, what if Zoe signed up for her 5K and got sick or had an injury that forced her to sit out? What should Zoe do? Should she bring up negative self-talk such as, "you're such a failure; you'll never reach your goals"? Should she spend the rest of her week angry at herself for her failure? Should she even call it a failure?

She shouldn't do any of these things. Instead, she should give herself a massive dose of compassion and embrace the fact that life is crazy-as-bananas. It's okay, the world is not coming to an end because she missed it. Her health is not going

After years away from running, I decided I wanted to get back into it again. To keep myself accountable, I volunteered to be a Girls-on-the-Run buddy. Being a mentor to fourth-grade girls ensured I showed up for the runs because I didn't want to leave them hanging. **–Zoe**

to tank because of it. She is going to be perfectly fine. It's easy to tell this to Zoe. The hard part is being able to say the same to yourself when you feel like you just flaked on a commitment. If you wouldn't say something to Zoe, then definitely don't say it to yourself.

This is why you'll hear me emphasize compassion over throughout this book. **Compassion is key.**

What if I don't have an activity that is impossible to flake?

Creating activities that are impossible to flake is a life practice. If you don't have one today, you will have opportunities in the future. Your task is to keep an open mind and watch for these opportunities when they come.

Your Assignment

PART ONE: *Pick an activity*

Write down one opportunity you have to create a scenario where exercise would be impossible to flake. Similar to the examples in the lesson, your opportunity will be completely unique to you.

My impossible-to-flake exercise: _____

If you already have exercise planned that is impossible to flake, it is okay to write these activities down.

PART TWO: *Your stress vs. reward*

Now, make an assessment of how much stress this will add to your week. Is the added stress worth the reward of the exercise and lifestyle? Does this enhance your life in the short or long term? Trust your gut instincts on this one. There is no right or wrong answer. This is your life, and you get to choose what will make you smile.

1. What additional stress does this impossible-to-flake exercise add to your life?

2. What can you do to help reduce the amount of stress this adds?

3. Is the additional stress of this impossible-to-flake activity worth the reward of exercise? Why or why not?

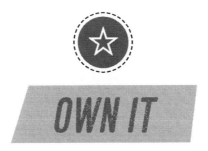

OWN IT

WEEK FIVE

Don't let others back-seat drive your life.

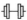

Exercise:

Go to Appendix C of this book and complete your exercise plans for Week 5.

Schedule your exercise plans into your calendar.

Lessons:

Your Success

Your Opinions

Your Heart

Your Time

Your Crazy Life

Your Healing

Your Sleep

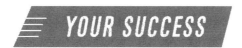
YOUR SUCCESS

It's time to quit giving your power away and start owning your success. We are going to let go of old excuses and push through with more speed than ever before.

LET'S DO THIS!

Own It—Your Success

You are developing an active lifestyle, and you want to do it in a way that brings happiness and health, not drudgery and injury.

IT'S TIME TO QUIT WISHING FOR IT AND START OWNING IT!

Own your exercise decisions. It's too easy to look around and compare your efforts to what others in your life are doing. There's a very good chance that most people in your life are sedentary and do not encourage you to get out and exercise. Don't make your success dependent upon their encouragement. Instead, own your success. Get out there and exercise even when nobody else is doing it. Get out there and exercise even on the days when nobody is watching you but you.

Empower yourself to do the type of exercise you like best. You do not need to let anyone push you into a specific program, especially if that program doesn't seem fun. Instead, take ownership—figure out what is fun for you.

If you're not sure what type of exercise you like, then own the responsibility of trying all kinds of activities until you find what you enjoy. Break through the stereotypes of who does what type of exercise, and keep an open mind. If the exercise you have chosen feels like another chore to cross off your list, it is doomed to fail. Take ownership of your success by not settling for anything less than something you enjoy.

Let's unpack this a little further. Not settling for anything less than something you enjoy does not mean you are going to immediately enjoy every form of exercise you do for a lifetime. You already know it isn't realistic to immediately enjoy every kind of exercise you ever do. In fact, for most of us, nothing is going to be "fun" in the beginning. It's going to suck to push your body into something it resists. Our bodies like homeostasis, which is a fancy way to say our bodies resist change. They prefer to conserve energy rather than expend it, and they naturally float toward relaxing rather than exercising. This principle is true for everyone, even elite athletes.

In this sense, owning your success means you commit to exercising regardless of whether you like it, and at the same time, you keep an eye out for other ways to exercise that are more enjoyable or more easily integrated into your life. Here's an example from Amy of how this played out in her life.

"I started jogging because it was the easiest cardio to do, not because I liked it. I felt like I was dying at first, and I never considered myself a 'runner.' Now, after almost 18 months, I'm almost a runner. I definitely like it more than I used to. I sometimes resist getting started, but I have to do that almost every day with every workout. BUT—the big change in me now is that I really do look forward to that feeling I get when I'm warmed up and hitting my stride during a run, and I really love the buzz after a good run. So yeah, I suppose it's finally 'fun' in that weird, warped, runner kind of way."

Amy spent more than a year doing an exercise she didn't love, but I believe that deep down she knew this was the right decision for her. She owned doing whatever it took to succeed, and took herself from sedentary to being able to run a sub-nine minute mile. Congratulations, Amy!

You can do the same by deciding up front if your aversion to an exercise is permanent or temporary. By owning your success, you also own deciding what type of exercise is right for you. If you blindly follow exercise routines that everyone else tells you to do, it won't bring you happiness and it won't last. When you are committed to owning your happiness and owning your decisions, this commitment transfers to every area of your life, including owning the type of exercise you choose.

You must relentlessly own your own success.

"I OWN MY SUCCESS. I AM EMPOWERED."

Let's take owning your success even one step further. It is misguided to believe that some day you will reach a perfect utopia of exercise bliss. I don't believe this perfection exists. Don't make the mistake of looking at athletes and assuming that their exercise journey is always on auto-pilot. It's not. Even the best of the best has ups and downs that never make it to a media headline.

I'd like to introduce you to someone who is among the best of the best—a man who holds 15 Guinness World Records, Erden Eruç (pronounced Air-den Air-rooch).

Erden became the first person in history to complete a solo human-powered circumnavigation of the globe. That means he traveled around the world with no motors, no sails, no engines whatsoever. He used his body, his mind, and his own muscle power to achieve what many thought was impossible. He rowed across the entire Pacific, Indian, and Atlantic Oceans solo; he biked, walked, jogged, kayaked, and covered a route that was 41,196 miles long. In addition to his amazing physical feats, he has an incredible wife, Nancy, whom he loves dearly. On paper, Erden has it all. But what the headlines don't share is how Erden fiercely battled the couch in his own unique way.

"When I returned to my home in Seattle, I was stuck on the couch, barely able to even move for six weeks. Here I was, an accomplished athlete with all these world records and all I could do was stare at the TV across the living room and my half-unpacked adventure gear. I was overwhelmed in a deep state of depression, and no, I couldn't just get over it.

"Nancy had moved to Sydney already having started a new job, and our plan all along was for me to join her as soon as possible, pack up the house and create a new life together in Australia. But instead, I spent the next six weeks alone in our home literally stuck on the couch. I knew she needed me there, and I truly wanted to be with her. I missed her presence—I wanted this change, and yet still, I was paralyzed by depression.

"My whole life had changed dramatically. Friends had moved on in their lives. Their children had grown. Life was similar for them, but life for me was forever changed. I did not see this coming. I felt alone and helpless, something I did not experience during my expedition. Even though I was alone, I had purpose and meaning. Now suddenly, the weight of the world was hanging on me like a dark cloud. Is this what real depression feels like, I wondered?

"Slowly and deliberately, and with the support of friends . . . with one tiny step at a time, I made my ascent. After four months, I was finally able to join Nancy. Yet the depression remained with me for a lot longer. Eventually I pulled myself back to the gym, back to being physical—a state I know so well. Exercise is where I feel like my old self. I forced my logical-self to rule over my emotions. One step at a time, and with professional help, I slowly found I could begin to rejoin life.

"I have great compassion and understanding for people who suffer from depression and also find themselves stuck on the couch. You are not alone! Support is out there. People do care and they want to help. But nobody can do this for you. It is possible to find hope and purpose again, and you will find many more moments of peace.

"Making a trip around the globe is kind of like getting unstuck from the couch. You can only conquer it one step at a time."

....

Erden's story is so incredible it's almost surreal, and yet the elements of his humanity apply to all of us. Since 2012 he achieved one more world record in rowing, and as I type this manuscript, Erden is in the middle of the Pacific Ocean on a sail boat as the Safety Officer for the Great Pacific Race, a biennial rowing race from Monterey Bay, California, to Honolulu, Hawaii. Erden achieved his latest world record in that very race in 2016, rowing this time with a partner. Outside of home, the ocean is where he feels most at peace.

It's now your turn to own the success in your life. Don't look to others to notice or congratulate you. That's not the point. You're not exercising for others. This is the one time it must be about you. You are creating the life you love, and only you get to decide what that looks like.

In today's assignment, you are going to begin a shift toward truly owning your success and not waiting for permission from others to live your life.

Start by reading this list of affirmations.

- *I am worthy of taking care of myself.*

- *I trust my intuition to guide me to the right exercise for me.*

- *I don't wait for others to give me permission to exercise.*

- *I don't wait for others to invite me to exercise with them.*

- *I don't make excuses or procrastinate.*

- *I'm compassionate toward myself.*

- *I take the next step needed.*

- *I am decisive.*

- *I am empowered.*

- *I am limitless.*

- *I own my success.*

Now, go back to the top of this list and read it through again.
This time think about which statement could have the greatest positive impact on your life if you began to practice it today. Circle that statement above.

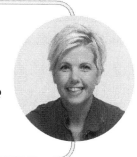

Your Assignment

Take your time when working through these questions.

1. On a scale of 1-10, how empowered do you feel today to own the decisions you make for your life?

1   2   3   4   5   6   7   8   9   10

2. Take a moment to reflect on your answer to question #1 above. Why did you choose this number as your answer for today?

3. How would your life look if you could improve that number?

4. How important is it to you to improve that number?

5. Why is it important to you to improve that number?

6. What is one action you can take this week to own your success?

Today, you are not going to solve all the world's problems. You are simply doing some thinking to get ready for the upcoming lessons.

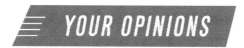
YOUR OPINIONS

The more opinionated you are about the benefits of exercise, the more likely you'll be to exercise.

Let's face it, most of us think about exercising every day but don't hold very strong opinions about the importance of how it helps your life today. You are going to start forming your own strong opinions about the immediate benefits in your life and in our nation. Having strong opinions about exercise will not only help you, it will help others around you. The more you take a strong stance on the importance of living an active lifestyle, the better chance we will have to inspire others to do the same. Together, we can lead a movement that trickles down to those around us and helps our entire nation become more active.

> **LET ME SAY IT ANOTHER WAY. BY HAVING STRONG OPINIONS ABOUT EXERCISE, YOU CAN HELP TAKE OUR NATION FROM COUCH TO ACTIVE.**

But first, you need to create your own strong opinions. Here are a few opinions to try on for size:

- **I am worthy:** *I truly believe that exercise is not a luxury and that I am worthy of having an active lifestyle. I no longer believe that exercise is a guilty pleasure.*

- **The status quo isn't good enough:** *Our sedentary lifestyles are not working. We are sicker than the generation before us. Health-care costs are rising, especially in the area of preventable disease. Exercise will help solve this national crisis.*

- **We all agree, but we still miss the mark:** *Everyone agrees that exercise is good for our health. We all have this elemental belief that exercise is good. Yet the vast majority of us miss the mark. We need to agree to put our beliefs into action.*

- **I can help our nation:** *I can help our nation's health-care crisis by exercising more and helping my friends do the same.*

- **No more exercise I hate:** *I want to live a life I love. I'm in this to increase the quality of my life. I'm no longer going to do exercise I hate. I'm going to figure out what's fun for me.*

- **I decide what type of exercise I love:** *I no longer need to cram myself into the box we typically think of for fitness. I'm here to be healthy, and that means all forms of exercise count.*

- **Exercise helps me to feel good every day:** *I'm not just chasing a distant goal, I'm enjoying the exercise I do each day.*

What are YOUR opinions on exercise?

By letting your opinions about exercise shine, you lead the way for others to do the same.

It's time to shine.

"MY OPINION COUNTS."

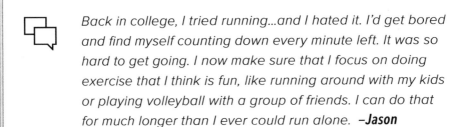

Back in college, I tried running...and I hated it. I'd get bored and find myself counting down every minute left. It was so hard to get going. I now make sure that I focus on doing exercise that I think is fun, like running around with my kids or playing volleyball with a group of friends. I can do that for much longer than I ever could run alone. **–Jason**

Your Assignment

PART ONE: *Get opinionated*

Create a list of opinions you have about the role of exercise in your life. What is important to you? What shifts do you need to make?

There are no wrong answers. Simply list what you feel strongly about. Make your list as long as you like, but be sure to list a minimum of five opinions.

1. _____

2. _____

3. _____

4. _____

5. _____

PART TWO: *Break a barrier*

Look at your **Breaking Barriers List** and pick one item you have a strong opinion about. It could be an opinion from the lesson above, or an entirely different opinion of your own. Spend a few extra minutes thinking about why it is important to you.

DO THIS WITH ONLY ONE ITEM IN YOUR LIST.

The barrier I feel strongly about:

This is my strong opinion about that barrier:

Holding this opinion is important to me because:

Again, we are not looking to solve everything at this point. We are gathering clarity on our barriers and seeing them in many different lights. By the end of the course, you will see how this groundwork plays into the bigger picture of your life as a whole.

BONUS ACTIVITY: SHARE!

To help solidify your opinions above, begin to share them with friends or family. However, there is one caveat to this activity: use wisdom as you share. I do not know what you have written down for your opinions, and I do not know your friends. I have no way of knowing if sharing these would actually be helpful to you. Use your own best judgment when sharing.

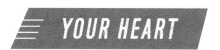

YOUR HEART

Who has the most influence over your heart?

GUESS WHAT?

That person wants you to exercise.

That's right, the very people you have sacrificed so much for—the very same people you have sacrificed your health for—want you to exercise. And yet, somehow, it's complicated.

Here's an excerpt from an article I wrote that shares a bit of how this played out in my life.

I have always loved biking. I don't care if I'm on the road or a backcountry trail. But I had a triple-whammy come my way. I have lung issues that are slowly eroding my cardiovascular strength. Asthma is one of those diseases that can be a total mind-#^@%. I spent years thinking, "oh, I just need to try harder." And when that didn't work, I spent years going to specialists in hopes of being able to heal my lungs enough to bike up that old hill without feeling like I have sandpaper rubbing the inside of my bronchial tubes. But I finally had to accept that my efforts haven't yet healed my lungs back to their old self. These days, I can no longer keep up with my friends on the bike. I need to go slower to protect my lungs. I have one loyal friend who is willing to ride with me at my snail's pace, and I haven't found "slow" friends to ride with yet. I'm not even sure if they exist.

I never gave up on biking. I never got lazy. Heck, I'm a certified cycle instructor. I have miles of single-track literally out the back door of my home. But those hilly trails I love have slowly grown into impassable mountains to me. Ever so slowly, the trails I love became out of reach for me. I've put on a few pounds. OK let's get real, I put on 20 pounds. This trajectory is freaking me out.

My body won't keep up with my spirit.

On a recent business trip, I called my hubby and told him how now, more than ever, I need to not give up on the hills in our neighborhood. I needed to figure out how to both continue to heal my lungs and ride my bike. I need to keep my chin up and bike however I can, even if it meant biking alone for now. I must keep smiling. I said these things knowing full well that realistically, I may never be able to ride those hills again. Ugh.

In comes the surprise.

When I came home from that business trip, I walked into my family room and saw a pedal-assisted electric bike with a bow on it. A gift for me.

I cried.

(A pedal-assisted bike has a silent electric motor to help make pedaling easier when you need it.)

It was one of those whirlwind moments when the emotions are all over the board. Sadness, because a pedal-assisted bike meant I had to accept that my hurting lungs need help. No more denial. Excitement, because I now could re-join my friends on bike rides instead of staying home alone. Love, because my hubby heard me and came up with this way to support me. Humbled, because I hadn't thought of it myself. Fear, because not everyone in the biking community is open-minded to bicycles that have a silent electric mini-motor attached.

I took all of those emotions, threw on my winter bike riding gear, and headed out the door. For the first time in years, I felt the freedom and joy of biking hills without an asthma attack leaving my chest in pain for days. I wasn't getting light-headed from a lack of oxygen, I wasn't the slow-poke holding everyone back, and I was getting a great workout.

It wasn't about the bike. It was about the freedom.

The freedom to get outside at a pace that is healthy for me, right now, today. The freedom to re-grow my physical strength in a way that brings me joy.

For this, I am more grateful than you know.

....

LOVE IS BOTH SIMPLE AND COMPLICATED.

My all time favorite quote on the topic of love is this.

> ### TO LOVE A PERSON IS TO LEARN THE SONG THAT IS IN THEIR HEART AND SING IT TO THEM WHEN THEY HAVE FORGOTTEN. –ARNE GARBORG

My husband knows my heart sings when I'm riding a bike with people I love. He sees me smile, thrive, and laugh. When biking turned into struggling with lung issues, he found a way to help me sing again. He saw me and heard me. He was truly a partner.

I also didn't make him guess. For years now I've been loving and clear about my needs, wants, and desires so he doesn't need to be a mind reader. I work hard to be the most supportive partner I can—likable, loving, and loyal. It's complicated and simple, all in one.

This isn't just for partners; it's for anyone in your life who has influence over your heart. Children, dear friends, and family all fit into this model. When you give someone a piece of your heart, you have also given that person the ability to influence how you spend your days and years. It's important that you carefully consider how impactful this is to your life as a whole. How much power are you giving them? Is it balanced or have you given away more than what is healthy?

Carefully consider the following questions as they apply to the people who have the most influence over your heart:

1. Does he/she know you have decided to have an active lifestyle?

2. How does that person know?

3. What can he/she do to be supportive?

4. How can you ask for help?

5. When will you ask for help?

6. Are you giving this person too much influence over you?

Your heart is where your courage is born. Magic begins when you realize that you have more support than you realized.

*After our heart-to-heart talk, my wife became my biggest supporter. I couldn't have done this without her. When I slowly helped her understand how important getting active was to me, I learned that she was always my best cheerleader. Now she knows how to support me even better. −**Jason***

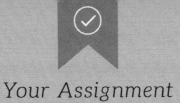

Your Assignment

PART ONE: *Your Heart*

List the people who have the most influence over your heart today. There are no wrong answers.

♡

MY HEART

1.

2.

3.

4.

5.

6.

7.

8.

9.

10.

11.

12.

13.

14.

PART TWO: *Reflections*

Below is the list of questions from our lesson. Carefully consider each question as it applies to your relationship with that person.

1. Does he/she know you have decided to have an active lifestyle?

2. How does that person know?

3. What can he/she do to be supportive?

4. How can you ask for help?

5. When will you ask for help?

6. Are you giving this person too much influence over you?

PART THREE: *Conversations*

Take five to ten minutes to carefully think through any conversations you need to have with the people in your list. Remember, they love you and want what is best for you. Sometimes, our loved ones just don't know what that looks like. We need to help them see the vision of your active lifestyle. This is not the place to whine, complain, or nag. You goal is to come to a place that is full of love and support.

KEEP IT SIMPLE.

Keep it full of love and kindness.

Remember, you are taking ownership of your success. They can help you, but your success is not dependent on their support.

Own your heart.

You've got this.

PART FOUR: *Your new life practice*

Yes, this is another life practice. From today forward, take ownership of your relationships with the people you love most by clearly communicating your needs to them with love and compassion.

"I communicate my needs, wants, and desires with love and compassion."

Remember that, deep down, your loved ones want what's best for you. By taking ownership of your needs and wants, you are becoming the best version of yourself. You are on your way to making this lifestyle change.

BONUS: Take another look at your **Breaking Barriers List**. Do you see any barriers where you can make progress by implementing this lesson?

TO LOVE A PERSON
IS TO LEARN THE SONG
THAT IS IN THEIR HEART
AND TO SING IT TO
THEM WHEN THEY HAVE
FORGOTTEN.

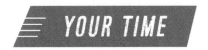

When it comes to exercise, I don't like time management quotes. How many of these platitudes have you been told multiple times?

- *"Nobody is too busy; it's a matter of priorities."*

- *"Either you run the day, or the day runs you."*

- *"Don't be busy, be productive."*

- *"Time management is life management."*

- *"We all have the same 24 hours in a day."*

Technically, every statement in the list above is true. But they're not helpful. Quotes like these may be the kick in the pants that gets us to take action in the moment, but they don't help us figure out how to get to the root issues controlling our time. **We need to dig deeper and make a breakthrough beyond this.**

You are already a high-achiever in many areas of your life. You have made personal sacrifices to be your best, and you have given your time away for the success of your career, your kids, your significant other, and a myriad of other priorities in your life.

However, reclaiming influence over your time can feel tricky. The people who influence your time don't always have your best interests at heart. For example, employers usually don't care if you exercise, and they might not see your health as something of their concern. I worked on many corporate projects that were excruciatingly demanding on my time. Over the years, I had several clients that sent me traveling for weeks at a time. Each long day started early and was followed by afternoon debrief sessions that wrapped directly into "optional" team dinners that went late into the evening. Working out in the morning only compounded the effects of jet lag and long-term sleep deprivation.

If you are a parent with young children, you could easily re-read the paragraph above and replace the references of clients and projects with babies and caregiving. The net effect is essentially the same. Sometimes we do have massive demands on our time. Family members may want you to exercise, but they may think of their needs as more important than yours, even when they don't say that directly to you.

So how do we even begin to make a breakthrough?

The Power of Predictability

When it comes to those who influence our time, we fall into patterns of predictability. We predictably get up at the same time, have a surprisingly predictable routine during the week, and even maintain a somewhat predictable routine each weekend. Your co-workers pretty much know when you show up, if you normally eat at your desk, and when you normally head home for the day. If you are home with kids, those beloved rug rats know you and your next step better than you realize.

This is not a bad thing at all. It takes energy to change a routine. Imagine if your routine changed every day. The change alone would be exhausting! Predictability is easier on the brain and brings a sense of peace.

However, right now, you need to make a shift to a new normal. You need to make exercise part of what is predictable about you.

MAKE EXERCISE PART OF WHAT IS PREDICTABLE ABOUT YOU.

Let's take the parent-child relationship. Part of the reason you feel no control over your time is because you have not taken control of your time. Now, stick with me here. I'm not talking about leaving your two-year-old home alone while you head to the gym. No, this is not remotely where we are going with this. I'm talking about making small subtle shifts that help you reclaim little pieces of your time. By slowly working through these shifts, your family will be able to adjust to the new normal, and it won't be so jarring to them. You'll no longer need to continue to sacrifice your health and pretend it's a joy.

For the corporate professional, you could read the paragraph above and replace the references to children with references to your work environment. It reads pretty much the same, doesn't it? You see, I'm not talking about quitting your job or letting the critical project fail. I'm talking about making small shifts that help you reclaim a more humane work environment. If you are struggling with an all-consuming job, you are not alone—your co-workers are struggling, too. There's just a tremendous amount of social pressure to appear like the daily grind of high-performance is a badge of honor.

Let's take a closer look at making this shift.

Making the Shift

Making the shift with your time is a sticky dance, and everyone's situation is unique. It's now time for you to be brave, own your time, and communicate your ownership to the people in your life who can influence your time.

When you first start this process, everything inside you is going to try to stop you. Fear is perfectly normal. Success comes when you push through the fear you have around truly owning your time. You need to take a leap of faith and remind yourself that fear is a state of mind. On the other side of this wall is the active lifestyle you are working so hard to gain.

Today, I am opening my heart and inviting you to view a dark corner of my past. Knowing I'm not alone gives me the courage to share.

"Owning my time used to be an impossible battle for me that I always lost. At the time, I didn't know my core issue was the fact that I didn't believe I was worthy of owning my time. I was blind to the self-deprecating space where I lived. If you asked me, I would have told you that I was strong and had huge responsibilities to uphold. I was a high-performing employee, a rock-star manager, a loving mother, and the sole provider for my home. I was terrible at doing anything for myself and a master at doing everyone else's bidding. Sometimes when I was particularly overwhelmed and desperate for a reprieve, I would have fantasies about breaking my leg or getting very sick just so I could have a 'valid' excuse to relax for a couple of weeks. I know in hindsight this is really messed up stuff. White-knuckling my way through life made me one tough cookie, but I wasn't remotely creating a life I loved. There was a level of misery immediately beneath my perma-smile because at my core, I didn't believe I was worthy."

You Are Worth It

Here is some food for thought to help you remember how attainable owning your time really is:

- *Right now, you can think of high-performing CEOs who are busier than you who still make exercise a priority.*

- *You know people who are busy and still exercise. Deep down, you have an added layer of respect for them. You also deserve to respect yourself in the same way.*

- *You actually can't really pinpoint where the fear of owning your time is coming from. If this is you, it's likely because it's new territory for you. The fear will go away once you cross this bridge.*

And remember our quote from the very first lesson in this book:

> *My body needs exercise.*
> *My body will always need exercise.*
> *This will never change.*
> *It's not negotiable, it's science.*

I'm not a big fan of using grit to motivate us to exercise. However, this particular lesson on owning your time will require you to muster up grit. It's far too easy for high-performing people to continue to let others rule their time. It's time for this unhealthy habit to change.

Let's summarize it all.

You need to let the people in your life who have influence over your time know that you have a renewed commitment to your health. Nobody can argue with living healthy. Sometimes we make the mistake of assuming we need to explain ourselves in detail or assure others that we won't fail in our duties. There's a good chance you don't need to give out these assurances. It's actually quite the opposite. Most of the time when you start doing a better job of owning your time, others in your life can relax knowing you've got your health managed as well as your obligations. And don't forget that your increased energy from exercise will help you get more done!

Start owning your time more, and many time management issues will work themselves out.

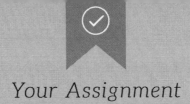

Your Assignment

PART ONE: *Your people*

Write the names of the people who have the most influence over your time today. This might be your boss, your children, or your partner or other family members. Many of the names will be the same as the previous lesson; there are no wrong answers.

YOUR PEOPLE

1.

2.

3.

4.

5.

6.

7.

8.

9.

10.

11.

12.

13.

14.

PART TWO: *Reflection*

Choose ONE name on your list.

Carefully consider each question as it applies to your relationship with that person and to owning your time.

1. Does he/she know you have decided to create an active lifestyle?

2. How does that person know?

3. Are you giving this person too much influence over how you spend your time?

4. What can you do today to begin to reclaim your time?

PART THREE: *Conversations*

Take five or ten minutes to carefully think through any conversations you need to have with this person. Remember, depending on the nature of the relationship, these conversations will probably look very different than the conversations you had in the previous lesson with your heart.

Keep it simple, upbeat, and positive.

Own your success. Your success is not dependent on this person's support.

PART FOUR: *Your new life practice*

Yes, this is another life practice: own your time.

From today forward, take ownership of your time and clearly communicate with the people who have influence over your time.

BONUS: Take another look at your **Breaking Barriers List**. Do you see any barriers where you can make progress by implementing this lesson?

YOU DO HAVE MORE POWER OVER YOUR TIME THAN YOU REALIZE. YOU ARE EMPOWERED.

YOUR CRAZY LIFE

You don't lack grit. You're not lazy. You simply have a crazy-as-bananas life.

Part of the reason you can't seem to find a "once and for all" solution to exercise is because it doesn't exist. Think of all the things in your life that make it a bit crazy. Do you really want them to all go away? Of course not. Do you aspire to have so little going on that you can rely on an exact exercise routine that is never interrupted? Do you want to be so rigid that you miss out on other amazing life opportunities that help you feel alive? I didn't think so.

Life is simply bananas, and for the most part, we like it that way.

Embrace Your Crazy Life

Guess what? Your exercise routines will always be changing. Today's exercise routines will be different six months from now, because your life is constantly changing—and that's how you want it. This wonderful life gives us challenges, trials, and gifts. It's all of the experiences combined that leave us in the end saying, "Yes! I lived!"

If we aren't diving in and surfing the crazy waves of life, we aren't living.

Please don't make a goal to have exercise 100% figured out for the rest of your life. Don't put yourself into a box where you quit having fun and are no longer creative with exercise. Don't ever find yourself doing the same exercises every week for years.

Exercise ebbs and flows with the waves of crazy that come our way—but we'll always return to our active lifestyles.

EMBRACE THE CRAZY.

Here are some examples of how people like you are embracing their lives.

"My kids are tremendous work, but I'm eternally grateful for their lives."

....

"Working full-time AND going to school at night is difficult, but it's my path to creating a life I love."

....

"My aging parent is ill and needs a lot of support, but I recognize that this is not forever, and this is part of the amazing circle of life."

....

"My house is always a mess, but this is because we are living and breathing."

....

"My job is exhausting me right now, but it provides for my family, and I am grateful for the talents and skills I have."

....

"I feel overwhelmed, but I'm doing better than I give myself credit for."

....

"Today, I just feel awful. That's okay. My life is not perfect. Nobody's life is perfect."

....

"I don't need to paste a smile onto everything. It's okay to be real."

....

CRAZY: IT'S ALL A PIECE OF THE BIG PICTURE.

You Need Balance

If your life is at a point right now where it is beyond crazy, or if you feel out of control, burnt out, mentally exhausted, and drained, then it's time to take a close survey of what's going on and think about how to improve your balance in the long run. While you work through this process, remember that the goal is for balance, not perfect control.

- *Are there physical shifts you need to make?*

- *Are there mindset adjustments you need to improve?*

- *Revisit the Breaking Barriers section of this book. Can you make a breakthrough?*

- *Do you need to go for a walk, relax, and think?*

We are all living this crazy, awesome, wonderful LIFE, looking at it in a new way, through a new lens. We are all doing our best to add physical activity so we can thrive in the crazy.

Life is bananas. It's also coconuts, grapes, apples, kiwi, cantaloupe, and mango. It's a big fruit salad!

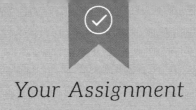

Your Assignment

PART ONE: *Your mindset*

Write several statements to help remind yourself that the craziness in your life is also part of living the life you love. You can use examples in the lesson to get started.

Mindset is everything when you have a full life with a lot of responsibility. When you are able create a mindset that rises above the chaos, you can see the big picture and remember that despite the craziness, you are living a life you love.

PART TWO: *Rebalance*

Are you completely out of balance? What should you do if you need to make a big change? What if your crazy life goes beyond a mindset shift and needs a big physical shift or a radical life change?

If this is you, hang onto those thoughts. We'll address these during the next set of lessons.

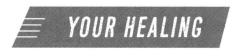

YOUR HEALING

Are you carrying around a backpack full of physical injury and mental strain? It can be difficult to look at these areas, but it's critically important to your growth. When you see the areas in your life that need attention, you can then begin the process of healing.

Has anything come up for you that needs healing?

Examples:

- **Physical:** *I need to figure out my back pain. I need to manage my foot pain better. I need to rein in bad eating habits and reach a healthy weight once and for all. I need to get my diabetes under control.*

- **Emotional/Mental:** *I need to manage my daily stress levels. I need to love myself more. I need to heal a relationship. I need space to breathe. I need to forgive someone. I need to ask for forgiveness. I need to better align how I spend my time with my true life priorities.*

REPEAT AFTER ME: I AM HEALING MYSELF.

You are not alone. All of us need some form of significant healing several times through our lives. If you think you don't, then knock on wood, because it happens. We all have areas where we need to heal and grow. Every single human on this planet has had challenges, failures, struggles, and trials. It doesn't make us any less human. Quite the opposite is true. The challenges we face in life are exactly what make us human. We're all in this crazy-as-bananas life together.

HEAL. DEFINITION: TO BECOME SOUND OR HEALTHY AGAIN.

If you've spent years or even decades relying on grit and ignoring areas that need healing, then it's a great opportunity to allow yourself room to breathe. If your aim is to be strong, you first need to heal. I know, you haven't purposely ignored tough areas in your life; you've just been preoccupied with the business of living. You've been pressing on in the name of strength while still carrying a very heavy load. It's time to take the heavy backpack you have been carrying, set it next to you, unpack it, and see if you can continue your journey with a lighter pack.

What is in your heavy backpack today? The good news is there is more support and less stigma around pretty much every aspect of healing people need today.

- **Physical healing:** *There's more science and data available now than ever to help people heal, and this is only going to get exponentially better over the coming years.*

- **Mental health:** *My heart smiles every time I see a dear friend be brave and share a mental health struggle. Finally, mental health has less stigma than ever before. It's about time.*

- **Emotional health:** *We understand more than ever about emotional intelligence and the importance of living with peace. The benefits of practices such as meditation are now being backed by science. There is emotional healing to be found.*

My goal is to inspire you to identify areas where you need to heal and then make a decision to find the support you need in order to heal.

HOW DO YOU NEED TO HEAL?

Imagine Healing

Imagine if you took the time right now to address areas of your life that need healing, both physical and emotional. How much more energy would you have for your active lifestyle? How much more joy would you feel day to day? How relieved would your loved ones be to see you becoming stronger because you are healed?

Being overweight for many years really did a number on my mindset. When I was finally completely honest with myself, I realized I was overcompensating at work to prove to myself that I was "good enough." My journey to live an active lifestyle is also allowing me to address some of those old mental and emotional wounds. I feel like the person I'm becoming is more whole and complete. **–Zoe**

My husband, Erik, has his own amazing story of healing. At the age of 21, he was diagnosed with rheumatoid arthritis. Gravity quite literally crushed him physically, mentally, and emotionally. Here's a small excerpt of his healing.

"The flare ups, exacerbated by work, left me disabled and barely able to walk. By age 30, I was a young man trapped in an old man's body. In a life spent escaping self-doubt, I had defined my sense of self-worth by what I could achieve physically. Now, as a young adult, my identity had eroded and my life was shrinking around me. Still, I doggedly denied my disability because I couldn't face the death of my identity.

"Then, it all flipped on its head when my orthopedic surgeon told me that total knee replacements were inevitable.

"Tears exploded out of my eyes like drops of water sizzling in a hot pan. The crushing finality of the doctor's proclamation snapped me out of my dogged denial that anything was wrong with me. It was devastating. Ten years of pain and uncertainty. The silent shame of pretending to be normal was exposed. RAW. Part of me was dead, gone forever. I don't know why I needed to hide from it, and who was I kidding? I'd been hobbling with a cane for six months.

"Through the surgery and bio-tech drug that healed me physically, I began to practice pushing through mental and emotional barriers that previously held me down. I got a second chance. This unlocked my soul and allowed me to explore life with a newfound freedom. Where could I go with such an escape from gravity?"

Like Erik, our areas that need healing tend to be important but not urgent, so they get pushed aside for years. But you can make a decision to change your trajectory today. Are you going to continue to rely on your grit and drive to carry burdens that instead could be healed? Or are you going to take the necessary steps to heal those wounds, whatever they are?

Yes, you are worthy of healing.
It's your decision.
It's within your control.
Own your healing.

Let me repeat myself: you are not going to heal everything today. You are, though, going to be inspired to heal and take your next step toward healing.

Remind yourself that exercise and physical activity have amazing healing properties. There is now a huge mountain of research that continues to support the importance of exercise as a way to improve our mental and emotional health. I know, you already know this.

Keep walking and keep moving as you stay committed to your healing.

Whew, I need to go for a walk....

"YES, YOU ARE WORTHY OF HEALING. OWN IT!"

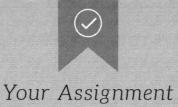

Your Assignment

PART ONE: *My healing list*

List the areas in your life where you need to begin or complete a healing process. There are no wrong answers and nothing is off-limits.

MY HEALING LIST

1. Physical healing

2. Emotional/Mental healing

3.

4.

5.

6.

7.

8.

9.

10.

11.

12.

13.

14.

PART TWO: *Start healing*

Look at your list again. Pick ONE item to begin to work on. Circle that ONE item and brainstorm what you can do to begin your healing.

1. What are your next steps for the ONE item you picked?

2. What is the date and time for the next step you will take toward healing?

Again, there are no wrong answers here. The only thing you can do incorrectly at this point is to NOT take action. If you don't know where to begin, then make a plan to start asking friends or research online. Whatever you do, don't give up. Your path will present itself.

PART THREE: *Your new life practice*

As time allows, commit to working on your entire healing list. Remember, life is always dynamic and changing. Your list of items that need healing will also change with time.

"I don't push my needs aside. I am healing myself."

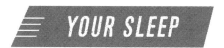

YOUR SLEEP

OUR GENERATION WAS WRONG.

So many of us were raised to think that sleep is for the weak. We were told that the ability to live on very little sleep meant we were strong, driven, and above the rest. In our youth, we wore all-nighters like a badge of honor, and in our middle years, we are proud of our knowledge of exotic coffee bean and energy drinks.

How well is this working out for us?

I'm glad to see a wave of research and books recently published on the topic of sleep and its importance. It has reinforced what we already know about sleep and exercise and validates sleep's importance to our "go hard or go home" generation.

We haven't always lived in a sleep-deprived manner. Did you know that, according to the National Institute of Health, most people in 1910 slept nine hours per night? But recent surveys show adults now sleep less than seven hours per night. The NIH estimates that sleep disorders affect as many as 70 million Americans. The Centers for Disease Control have some fascinating data graphs showing the amount of sleep deprivation plotted on a map of the United States.

ALMOST HALF OF US ARE LITERALLY YAWNING OUR WAY THROUGH LIFE.

Sleep helps our bodies recover from exercise and aids motivation to exercise in the first place. It influences body weight, heart health, mental acuity—pretty much everything hinges on getting enough quality sleep.

The list of what we know about sleep continues to grow. Sleep:

- *Balances growth and stress hormones;*

- *Supports the immune system;*

- *Decreases risk of obesity, heart disease, and infections;*

- *Aids in cellular repair; and*

- *Boosts our ability to think creatively.*

Thankfully, we have finally come full circle and again recognize that sleep is not for the weak; it's for the strongest among us.

SLEEP: IT'S NOT OVERRATED.

My early 30s was the pinnacle of my sleep deprivation story. I had an entire winter where I didn't once sleep more than four hours straight. Daily minimums included three shots of espresso, which is easy to do living in Seattle. My high-adrenaline job at a start-up firm kept me believing I was alert. Every winter I got sick and shrugged it off as normal. Blood-shot eyes were chalked up to getting old. I ignored the signs of exhaustion because my VP and clients were happy. However, looking back, I realize that my lack of energy kept me from seeing creative ways to break free from this unhealthy environment. It wasn't until my sleep improved that I had the mental space to make a breakthrough—the breakthrough that led me to create COUCH to ACTIVE. I believe that if I had never made a breakthrough with my sleep, I wouldn't be where I am today. Sleep helped me see opportunities. Sleep leveled up my game.

SLEEP HELPED ME SEE OPPORTUNITIES. SLEEP LEVELED UP MY GAME.

I want you to also level-up your ability to see opportunities in your life and make a breakthrough.

Sleep and Opportunities

For today's lesson, we are going to use what we know about the benefits of sleep to sharpen our ability to SEE OPPORTUNITIES to exercise. When coming up with solutions for our active lifestyle, we need to be creative, break barriers, see mini-solutions, and jump on these opportunities when we see them. After all of the research that has come about with sleep and people's ability to problem solve, we must use sleep as another one of our tools to break through barriers to fitness. Getting rested is going to help us do this.

SLEEP IS GOING TO HELP US CREATIVELY PROBLEM SOLVE.

Our goal is to live a life where regular, quality sleep is normal. This is our guiding principle. However, in reality, most of us are over-achievers who live an incredibly full life that borders on overcommitted. So, with this in mind, we are going to give ourselves an additional tool that will help us identify when we need to make a radical change.

Knowing we should get eight hours of sleep is just the beginning. We also have to look at habits that interfere with our ability to get that sleep. Many of us are doing a salsa dance with caffeine and alcohol. We caffeinate to wake up in the morning and use alcohol in the afternoon to buffer from the day's stress. We end our day with alcohol in the hope it will lull us to sleep.

It's not just lifestyle that causes sleep issues. Sleep apnea, stress, anxiety, joint pain, fibromyalgia, and a whole host of factors can interfere with our sleep. The lack of sleep can compound your health issue. If you are experiencing any of these, head back to our lesson on Healing and give yourself the gift of working through these health issues. Not all health issues are solvable, but most are manageable. You deserve it, and you are worthy.

Sleep issues can easily become our number one barrier to exercise, but exercise can also be part of the answer to many sleep issues. Many health issues make exercise harder to do, but exercise can also improve or heal those health issues. In this case of the chicken or the egg, exercise must always come first.

Being the primary caregiver for my kids, I'm used to being sleep-deprived. I pushed through, telling myself it was a normal part of parenting. But, as I got less and less sleep, my energy levels took a nosedive, my mind was foggy, and the numbers on the bathroom scale steadily crept up. I'd wake up each morning feeling barely able to function and would use my daily two or three cups of coffee to get me going. Then by the afternoon, I'd have my own happy hour in the kitchen while cooking dinner. Over the course of a couple of years, the one-drink happy hour had slowly slipped to sipping red wine through dinner followed by a night cap to help me sleep. The alcohol messed with my sleep, which left me dragging even more in the morning. For me to make sleep a priority, I had to also manage alcohol and caffeine's role in my life. Once I worked through that, I had more energy to share with my wife and kids, and I'm not constantly forgetting things like I used to. **–Jason**

The Three-Day Sleep Test

It's time to give yourself the Three-Day Sleep Test. Each month, look at your calendar and find three days in a row where you have a chance to get a minimum of eight hours of sleep. Then protect those days and get the rest. After about three days of rest, you'll notice you can think more clearly, and everything seems easier to manage.

The practice of checking in on opportunities to sleep is a meter you will use to evaluate if your life truly is out of balance and you need to make a radical change.

There are no exceptions to this three-day rule. You are a human, and all humans need sleep. It doesn't matter if you're busy at work or if you are a new parent. Every human needs sleep. However, there are seasons in our lives where consistent sleep is impossible and the choice to sacrifice sleep is the right decision. If you are in one of those seasons, give yourself a big dose of compassion and recognize it as a temporary phase in your life that you intend to improve at a future date.

OWN YOUR SLEEP.

If You Can't Sleep

If you suffer from insomnia, sleep apnea, or any other health issues that interrupt your sleep, please give yourself a massive dose of compassion. You already know that a lack of sleep impacts your life, and I don't want this lesson to add stress to your day. The three-day rule can still work to your advantage.

If the paragraph above describes you, take the three-day rule and simply rest quietly in your room for the eight hours. Don't worry about actually sleeping—just find three days that you can devote eight or more hours of rest time in your own bed with no TV, phone, or other screens to keep you awake. While you are resting, your brain will continue to process your day. During this time, your brain will help you be creative, break barriers, and see mini-solutions so you can jump on them.

Your Assignment

It's time to begin your new life practice around sleep. Do this life practice every month.

PART ONE: *Take the Three-Day Sleep Test*

1. Open your calendar now and pick three days in a row to sleep a minimum of eight hours. You must find the three days sometime within the next four weeks.

2. Create a calendar reminder for the three days of quality sleep and protect those days.

PART TWO: *Evaluate for red flags*

Obviously, our greater goal is to have consistent sleep every night. We know this. However, for the purposes this assignment, focus on the three-day test as a means to identify if you are completely out of balance and at risk of losing health or work performance as a result of your continual lack of sleep.

If on any given month you cannot find three consecutive days to sleep for a minimum of eight hours, then you need to flag this as an issue and look at how to resolve it.

PART THREE: *Other factors*

1. Is caffeine getting in the way of healthy sleep habits? If yes, what can you do today to start to resolve this issue?

2. Is alcohol getting in the way of healthy sleep habits? If yes, don't delay—take immediate charge of your alcohol consumption. Alcohol is relentless. It doesn't care if you are the nicest or smartest person in the room. What can you do today to work toward resolving this issue?

3. Do you have health issues that are getting in the way of your sleep? What can you do today to continue to work through these issues?

4. Do you have a permanent health issue or other lifestyle factor that you cannot influence today? If so, have compassion. We will address permanent barriers in upcoming chapters.

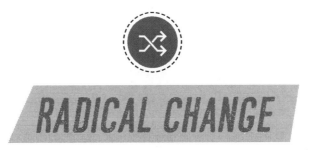

RADICAL CHANGE

Week Six

Are you stuck?

Exercise:

Go to Appendix C of this book and complete your exercise plans for Week 6.

Schedule your exercise plans into your calendar.

Lessons:

You Are in Control

Are You Stuck?

Being Brave

Barriers to Stay

YOU ARE IN CONTROL

If you've made it this far and still feel stuck, don't lose hope. There is a good chance you are facing bigger challenges than you realized, and you might need to make a huge decision to transform your life. In the next few chapters, you will get clarity on the items in your life that need a radical change.

THE STRUGGLE IS REAL.

If the thought of making a radical change in your life triggers stress, if you have a pit in your stomach just reading this, then your assignment is to take a long walk and breathe. Remind yourself that you are the one in control of your life and your decisions. You choose what to do next. Nobody can make you do anything you do not want to do or anything you are not ready for.

On the other hand, maybe you're the one holding yourself back. You are the one who has to make the decision to step forward. Most of the time, we already know what we need to do to improve our lives, and taking the next step forward can be as simple as deciding to make the change rather than continuing to sit on it. I want you to be brave and bold, but you have to want it more than I do. Ultimately, the choice is yours. It's your life.

YOU ARE EMPOWERED.

The good news is that when you feel completely stuck, it means you haven't given up on your dream to make a breakthrough. It means there's still hope.

Massive frustration is where radical changes begin.

FRUSTRATED? GOOD, YOU HAVE NOT GIVEN UP YET.

Ponder the idea that you may need to make a radical change in your life. If this is you, take a moment to open yourself up to the possibility of great changes ahead.

In upcoming chapters, you are going to accomplish the following:

1. You will get crystal clear on the areas in your life where you feel stuck.

2. You will recognize the difference between feeling stuck and making a decision for change.

3. You will identify the areas where you are going to make radical changes.

4. You will strengthen your ability to be brave in the face of change.

5. You will decide where you are not going to make a radical change, and instead work toward finding happiness despite the existing challenge.

    This could be a crossroads in your life.

LET'S GET STARTED.

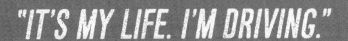

Your Assignment

There is no written assignment for this lesson.

Instead, take a few minutes and go for a walk outside. Breathe the fresh air and remind yourself of the progress you have made so far.

I hate to admit this, but as the primary caregiver for my kids, there are times that I feel completely overwhelmed and out of control. But how can I possibly admit I need help? At times, I feel like my kids are controlling my life, and if my wife's working long hours, I don't have the backup and support I need. On those days, I really do feel like I am going to lose my mind. **–Jason**

ARE YOU STUCK?

All the life practices and routines in the world will ultimately fail if we haven't addressed barriers that need radical change.

In this lesson, you are going to identify any areas in your life where you are stuck and need radical change.

Below are examples of common areas where people get stuck. Each example includes a trigger point. Use the trigger point to help you identify if this is an area in your life where you might also be stuck.

Your Job—*Trigger point*—You're driving to work dreading each day, you're unhappy all day, you watch the clock until it's time to go home, and you can't wait for the weekend. It's draining your energy, which makes exercise feel impossible.

Your kids or aging parents—*Trigger point*—You have no backup or nobody to cover for you so you can do anything on your own. You feel totally overwhelmed, and you find yourself begging the universe for a five-minute break.

Your extra commitments—*This is a tricky one.* Once we have publicly made a commitment, it's difficult for our brain to let it go, even if we know it's the best thing for us. Maybe you know you need to let go of an extra commitment. ***Trigger point*—**You find it very difficult to say no. You are harboring resentment toward a commitment you currently hold.

Your physical limitations—*This could be short-term or long-term.* If it's lifelong, then your job is to take radical steps to get the adaptive equipment you need. It can require a radical commitment and time, but you can get yourself unstuck. ***Trigger point*—**you are physically unable to exercise a minimum of 30 minutes five days a week.

Your mental or emotional challenges I'm so glad to see our society beginning to de-stigmatize mental health issues. The challenges are real; when we ignore them and don't get help, we stay stuck. ***Trigger point*—**You have a daily sense of unease about life. If in doubt, seek support without delay.

Your big-deal life events—*This one takes all shapes and forms.* Job changes, layoffs, newborns, moving to a new city, tragedies, marriages, divorces, abusive relationships, surgeries, working through addiction issues, or even winning the lottery are all "big-deal" life events.. Most of these upset the whole cart and require a full reset through all the life practices in this book to get back to a healthy normal. For each of these areas, give yourself a full month of compassion to process the issue. ***Trigger point*—**After a month, if you are still not back to your active lifestyle, this is your flag that it's time to revisit the life practices.

IS IT POSSIBLE TO HAVE A TIME IN YOUR LIFE WHEN YOU ARE STUCK AND NOT EXERCISING IS THE RIGHT DECISION?

Yes, this is quite possible. If you've worked through all of the lessons on breaking barriers, you've exhausted all resources available to you, and you are truly stuck, setting consistent exercise aside might be the right decision for a short period in your life.

I want to stand here and maintain that there is always a way to exercise through every single phase of your life, 100% of the time. We can use mini-solutions, we can recruit our friends, we can set boundaries, and we can make an exercise commitment impossible to flake. However, it is possible that life can honestly throw us a huge curve ball where exercise lands in the back seat for a while.

This is a very personal choice based on very extenuating circumstances.

My dear friend Amy Rosendahl had a "big-deal event" that put most exercise on hold. Her partner, Joe Stone, was in a tragic accident and suffered a spinal injury that left him an incomplete C7 quadriplegic. Here's a piece of Amy's story:

> *"I had just the month prior completed my very first marathon. This was completely a couch to marathon experience for me. It was amazing because I had just found a whole new level of fitness for myself, and then my partner had a really horrific and terrible accident. He was speed flying, which is kind of like paragliding, and crashed. His injuries were so significant he really should have died. He was in a drug-induced coma for a month and was in the hospital for four months. I went from 'Oh my gosh, I can run a marathon; I can do anything!' to sitting next to a hospital bed for four months. For the first part I was just hoping he lived, and the second part I was helping him rehab, helping him eat, brush his teeth, and go to the bathroom. All of the little things consumed my life.*
>
> *"When I was going through that time in my life, I wanted to exercise. The plan after my marathon was to keep it going. The marathon was my*

first big physical accomplishment. But it was so hard. When I wasn't at work, I was sitting next to his hospital bed. But not being by Joe's side gave me a lot of anxiety, so I decided that not exercising for that time in my life was the right thing to do. For about eight months, I was pretty much sedentary. I joined a gym with hopes of that motivating me. But the motivation has to come from inside yourself, and I didn't get there often. Contrary to what some might wrongly assume, I was still making myself a priority. I prioritized my mental health over exercise so I could be there for Joe. This was exactly where I needed to be, and I don't regret that at all. No regrets, no regrets at all."

Amy is currently a three-time Ironman finisher! That's right, 2.4-mile swim, 112-mile bike ride, and a full marathon. Amy didn't just find her way back to an active lifestyle, she made her way back to the elites. Way to go, Amy!

Joe Stone also has his own amazing recovery story. He is now one of a handful of wheelchair users in the world to pioneer adaptive paragliding. He recently earned his P3 rating, and he explores new sites regularly. He is most certainly pushing the envelope of adaptive free flight.

If you find yourself in a position similar to Amy's, where exercise must take a back seat, it really is okay. Like Amy, having a unique period in your life where exercise takes a back seat does not mean all hope is lost. It doesn't mean you'll never find your way back to an active lifestyle. Never give up hope, and you will find your way back to an active lifestyle.

The bad news about being stuck is that your body still needs exercise. So make any decision to take a break from exercise with much compassion and caution. Own your decision, and don't fall into negative self-talk that will only increase your stress over your current situation.

In the next few lessons, we are going to dive deeper and unpack what to do when we are stuck so that we can maintain a healthy frame of mind and work our way back to an active lifestyle.

OWN IT: You're stuck, and you're going to work your way out.

Your Assignment

List any areas where you are stuck.

- Your job
- Your kids or aging parents
- Your outside commitments
- Your physical limitations
- Your mental or emotional challenges
- Your "big-deal" events

AM I STUCK?

AREAS I AM STUCK:

1. My job is sucking the life out of me.

2. I have no backup support for my kids.

3. I'm struggling with depression.

4.

5.

6.

7.

8.

9.

10.

11.

12.

13.

In the following lesson, you will take a closer look at each item you listed above and decide if you are going to take action now, later, or never.

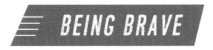

BEING BRAVE

IT'S DECISION TIME.

You are now going to make strategic decisions on which of your barriers are here to stay and which you intend to resolve.

You are going to become crystal clear on each of your barriers from the previous lesson by labeling each item in one of these categories:

1. **Radical Change.**
   You are going to take steps toward resolving this barrier in your life. You may not know exactly what to do or where to start, but you are going to begin the path.

2. **Permanent, no change possible.**
   This is a permanent item that will not change in your lifetime.

3. **Deferred.**
   Change is possible. You plan to resolve this eventually, but you are choosing to NOT take steps toward resolution today.

Once you work through this process, you will have more clarity over how you will approach each of your big barriers. Having this clarity will help you focus your energies on efficiently breaking barriers rather than staying stuck in the overwhelm. Your brain will be able to relax a little and focus on what is important.

You must be brave and advocate for yourself. There will always be moments of self-doubt. Your brain is naturally wired to resist change and keep you where you are. Be sure you don't overthink this process at the expense of pushing through to the change you need. If you find your brain trying to hold you back with fear, pause and remind yourself that you are in charge of your life. Fear is not your boss. You are empowered to continue with the direction you have chosen.

If you find yourself feeling stuck and wanting to overthink areas you have deferred, again remind your brain that you made the decision to defer these for now. It is okay to let some items rest.

No more fear-based decisions.

IT'S TIME TO BE BRAVE.

Bravery is not the lack of fear, but the ability to move forward in spite of the fear. The changes you make become more important than the fear you experience. There will always be fear. We all have fear. I have fear every single time I do something new and work toward the next breakthrough in my own life. There isn't a single human on this planet who is immune to fear.

Fear is a normal feature that is designed to keep you safe. It tells you to run away from tigers, avoid raging rivers, and keep your hands out of fires. However, in today's relatively safe world, most of our fear arises when we face changes, perceive threats to our own egos, or risk disappointing someone.

The emotion of fear can feel so strong that we have a difficult time seeing that there is actually nothing valid to fear. Fear keeps us from jumping in front of a car when crossing a road or eating sushi leftovers that sat out all night. This is good fear. On the other hand, the fear of looking bad in Spandex is different. The fear of people wrinkling their noses at you because you are taking care of yourself is different. Never making the change you so badly need because you are afraid you might offend someone is different. You get my point. You are not going to die; you are actually on the path toward thriving. You are worthy of this healthy lifestyle, and pushing past your fears is required to make the change.

When you recognize your fear as an emotion you can push through, taking your first step becomes easier.

In addition to fear, part of what keeps us stuck is not having clarity on how our lack of action impacts our lives today and in the future. This is especially true with difficult decisions or decisions that will impact others in our lives.

LET ME SAY THAT AGAIN: Lack of action also has consequences.

Here's a tool that I use that will help you decide which areas in your life need radical change and which areas you are not going to change at all or defer for the future. I work through this list of questions to help bring clarity.

1. How much does this impact you physically?

2. How much does this impact you emotionally?

3. How often is this on your mind?

4. Why is this on your mind?

5. Why is this important to you?

6. Dig even deeper. Take your answer to question #5 and ask yourself why that answer is important to you today.

7. Dig even deeper. Take your answer to question #6 above and ask yourself why that answer is important to you today.

8. How will your life improve if you resolve this?

9. What will happen if you don't resolve this?

10. What can you do to be brave?

Don't apologize for who you are becoming. Create your own life. Stand up tall and own it. It all starts with being brave.

Not too long ago, I was really struggling with my job. My team was working on a proposal for a potentially huge deal with a client, and my work-life balance was nonexistent. I was missing out on sleep, exercise, and just about everything that kept me healthy. The physical stress was hurting my emotional well-being and keeping me from being present for my family. I wanted to show up as a better partner for my husband and to be the one who brought joy back into our relationship. I didn't want to continue down the slippery slope of my worn-out crabby state, and I was honestly afraid our marriage might not survive at this pace. I had to sit down and do some serious thinking about how I could delegate some tasks or carve out time to take care of myself. **–Zoe**

"DON'T APOLOGIZE
FOR WHO
YOU ARE BECOMING."

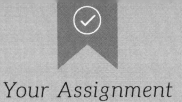

Your Assignment

PART ONE: *Take ownership*

Take a look at the previous lesson where you listed areas where you felt stuck. Take each item one at a time and answer these questions from our lesson. There's enough room here to work through one item. You may need to use the extra notes pages at the back of this book to work through additional items.

1. How does this impact you physically?

2. How does this impact you emotionally/mentally?

3. How often is this on your mind?

4. Why is this on your mind?

5. Why is this important to you?

6. Dig even deeper. Take your answer to question #5 and ask yourself why that answer is important to you today.

7. Dig even deeper again. Take your answer to question #6 and ask yourself why that answer is important to you today.

8. How will your life improve if you resolve this?

9. What will happen if you don't resolve this?

10. Can you be brave?

PART TWO: *Decision Time*

Now you are going to give each item a decision for today. This is where you are going to begin to get unstuck.

TAKE ANOTHER LOOK AT YOUR LIST FROM THE PREVIOUS LESSON.

Next, place each item into one of these categories. Write the category title next to each item.

1. Radical Change.

2. Permanent, no change possible.

3. Deferred.

You now have more clarity over which items you will focus on and which items you are choosing to let rest for now. Having this clarity will help you focus your energies on efficiently breaking barriers rather than staying stuck in the overwhelm.

For the items you labeled "Radical Change," take a moment to think of the next action step you need to take for that item. Don't delay, start taking action today. For many reading this book, these items are huge, and your first step will be to seek help. This is a perfectly valid first step.

For today, simply commit to seeking out your answers and being brave as the path reveals itself to you. In our next lesson, you'll take a closer look at what to do with the items in your list that are permanent or deferred.

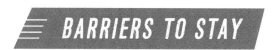

BARRIERS TO STAY

You've decided a barrier is here to stay. Now what?

Now your task is to work toward having a healthy frame of mind for these sticky barriers that aren't going away anytime soon. The purpose of this is to be in a place of owning your life rather than reacting to it.

IT'S NO SURPRISE THAT THIS IS MUCH EASIER SAID THAN DONE.

The first step is to reframe how you talk to yourself about these barriers. I'm not asking you to put on your rosy glasses or dive into a pit of self-denial. And I'm definitely not telling you to just "suck it up, Buttercup." The barriers you are facing are real, the frustration is real, and when faced with a barrier where there is no immediate fix, the best thing you can do is to get your mindset about that barrier into a space that eases the amount of mental distress it causes you. When you reduce the stress you have over things you can't control, you also begin to see each barrier more objectively.

Below is the thought process that will help you begin to find your healthy frame of mind.

- *This barrier will remain in place because...*

- *I aim to work on this barrier when...*

- *I will not let it sabotage my active lifestyle by...*

- *I'm grateful because...*

- *I will show myself compassion by...*

Here are a few examples of how this plays out.

A Stressful Job: I've been dreading and hating my job for a couple of years. For today, this barrier is going to stay in place because I need the income and don't have the option to quit without another job. I am going to work on getting a new job; my first step is to develop the skills I need for a career I enjoy more. I will not let this job sabotage my active lifestyle; instead, I will use two lunch breaks a week to exercise. I also think I can leave a bit early on Fridays to exercise. I'm grateful for this job. It provides for my needs, and it's giving me good work experience. As a bonus, I have a made a couple of friends at work. I'm going to show myself compassion by getting up early enough in the morning to not be rushed. I'm also going to do my very best work. I might hate my job, but I'm going to take pride in my work because that is the kind of person I want to be.

....

__A Big-Deal Event:__ I just broke my leg in a car accident. I obviously can't make this go away, and it's impacting my ability to exercise in a big way. I'm not going to let it sabotage my active lifestyle, because I will figure out what kind of exercise I can do, no matter how small or insignificant it may feel. I'm also going to look at my normal eating habits and ensure I eat healthy and eat a little less. This will help me feel good and gain less weight in the healing process. I'm grateful I wasn't hurt worse. I am going to show myself compassion every day by giving myself extra time to get places and asking friends for help. I may even have groceries delivered or allow myself more takeout for a few weeks. I'm also going to invite friends over to hang out, and I won't worry about how much of a mess the house has become.

....

__Extra commitments.__ I'm overcommitted with volunteering at my kids' school. I've become resentful of the work, and I know I need to let this go. But I'm in the middle of the school year and have decided that I want to keep my commitment for the year. So for now, this barrier is going to stay. I am going to let the school know that this will be my last year as chair, and I won't let them talk me out of the decision. In the meantime, I will not let it sabotage my active lifestyle by doing my best to simplify the current commitments I have made. I'm incredibly grateful for my children and the school community; they are big parts of my vitality. I am going to show myself compassion by reminding myself this is my last year and by not allowing myself to be sucked into being the chair again next year.

....

__Permanent health issue.__ I have asthma; this likely will not change for *the rest of my life. I am committed to listening carefully to my body and avoiding asthma triggers. This will help to keep me as healthy as possible. I'm not going to let asthma sabotage my active lifestyle. Instead, I will get massively creative and look for ways to be active that are right for me. I'm grateful for everything I can do and that I live in a climate that lets me get outside most days. I'll show myself compassion by pausing when I catch myself feeling negative about my asthma and how it holds me back. I will quit the comparison game and instead strive to be an inspiration to others by my example of working with this difficult health issue. I'll also look for new friends who are more at my fitness level.*

Mindset is everything when it comes to barriers that are here to stay. A healthy mindset can be exactly what keeps us from giving up on the active lifestyle that we want so badly.

Anne has been through barriers that would crush the average person. She's a talented middle school teacher and theater director who has faced tremendous barriers to exercise. She is dealing with complications from a surgery that resulted in multiple follow-on hernia repairs, gastric sleeve surgery, and even more surgery to come. Anne knows what it's like to have barriers that are here to stay. I'll let her share a piece of her story.

"This past month the pain has slowly gotten worse, and I am having to accept the fact that it has been almost two years and this chronic pain is not going away anytime soon. My life is significantly different than it was two years ago. I had to quit my job, remove all exercise, and avoid any strenuous activities. Heck, even standing or sitting too long can be too much, and don't even make me laugh when I am in pain.

"Slowing down has hurt me physically and been mentally challenging. Most days I need to spend hours just laying flat. If I do anything even as simple as cooking a dinner, I have to lay down afterwards. Shopping is becoming impossible. I ask myself how I can be a mother when I can't do the job without pain? Cleaning is impossible, and not being able to do physical activities with my kids breaks my heart. While I type this my whole family is out on a gorgeous hike, and I am once again cooped up in the house.

"I now have more compassion than ever for people who deal with chronic pain—because I am one of them. When you see me, I do my best

to be full of smiles because I want so badly to experience glimpses of what my normal life used to be. What you may not realize is that for that portion of the day I am good, but I will be in bed paying for it later. I have days where I feel good, only to wake up the next morning wondering if I can make it out of bed. It is hard not to dwell on it, or let the pain push me toward depression.

"I may be physically stuck, but I am still a smiler, I am a laugher, and I am a social butterfly. So I will suck it up, refuse to let this beat me, and go about my day.

"I have another surgery on the horizon that I hope will heal my pain. Between now and then, I'm doing the very best I can to show myself compassion and remind myself I am still valuable with or without my health issues. My goal right now is even with the pain to get out and walk around my block with my hubby each night. It makes a world of difference even doing that one small thing.

"People ask me how they can help. Pray, pray for healing, pray for wisdom and guidance. Be an encourager. And please, don't judge my messy house. :)"

....

Anne is an amazing woman. She continues to impress me by what she can accomplish despite the significant challenges she faces. I am also looking forward to the day when Anne is fully healed and her body can finally keep up with her beautiful and bright spirit.

We all experience major life changes that present significant barriers to exercise. With this tool, you can begin to break out of feeling stuck and instead have the confidence that you have chosen your current path for valid reasons.

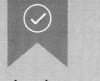

Your Assignment

It's your turn to write your paragraphs about the barriers that are deferred or here to stay.

WRITE YOUR OWN PARAGRAPHS FOR YOUR TOP BARRIERS THAT ARE HERE TO STAY.

Your goal is to find a healthier frame of mind that will help you live with more peace and confidence that the barrier will not beat you down.

Below is space to work through one barrier. Use the blank notes pages at the back of the book to complete additional items.

My barrier that is here to stay: _____

This barrier will remain in place because...

I aim to work on this barrier when...

I will aim to not let it sabotage my active lifestyle by...

I'm grateful because...

I will show myself compassion by...

YOUR NEXT TWO YEARS

WEEK SEVEN

Stay on track with a rock-solid plan.

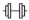

Exercise:

Go to Appendix C of this book and complete your exercise plans for Week 7.

Schedule your exercise plans into your calendar.

Lessons:

Blink

Magic Takes Time

Holidays and Events

Two More Years

Escape a Setback

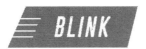

What's next month going to look like for you?

BLINK!
ANOTHER MONTH HAS GONE BY.

How will the rest of your year play out?

BLINK!
ANOTHER YEAR.
BLINK–BLINK...

Think back to the past six weeks. In some respects, you probably feel like you've been working through this book forever. In other ways, you feel like you've just begun. Regardless, you've made tremendous progress in a short amount of time.

Time flies. Think about where you were exactly two years ago. What's the same? What's different? How fast did the last two years fly by?

Let me repeat that:
HOW FAST DID THE LAST TWO YEARS FLY BY?

Your next two years are going to fly by even faster.

Let's say that again too:
YOUR NEXT TWO YEARS ARE GOING TO FLY BY EVEN FASTER.

If you stop your progress here, you will slide back to your sedentary lifestyle. When life throws you a curveball, you might not ever get back to your active lifestyle. I know you don't want this to happen.

This is why you are going to work through your own two-year plan.

Your two-year plan will enable you to take charge of the coming weeks. You'll have the framework to make the very MOST of your growth with the very LEAST amount of added time to your year.

You will not just have an active lifestyle; you will have clarity on how you got there, and you will know exactly what to do to get back on track when life throws you a curveball.

You are now truly owning it!

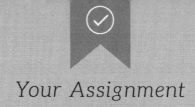

Your Assignment

There is no written assignment for this lesson.

TAKE A FEW MINUTES TO CAREFULLY PONDER THE IDEAS BELOW.

PONDER THIS

Take a moment and breathe.

Let the idea of how fast time flies sink in.

Imagine your next two years. Imagine the sense of urgency around taking ownership of the upcoming days, weeks, and years.

Commit to yourself today to NOT BLINK. Instead, you are going to make the very most of your next two years to let your changes grow into a new lifestyle.

MAGIC TAKES TIME

It's usually not too difficult to integrate a new habit into our lives when our schedules are predictable and smooth sailing. In theory, a predictable schedule sounds great, but unfortunately, it's completely unrealistic. This is especially true around holidays, vacations, and any other special event that throws off our schedules. Fortunately, we can see many of these events coming before they hit. We know that each year we celebrate certain holidays, we have family members with birthdays, and many of our jobs have annual retreats or events planned out months in advance.

Knowing about all of these events ahead of time is good, because it means we can also plan ahead and integrate each one into our active lifestyles. We can proactively plan for holidays, annual events, and other days that typically get in the way of exercise. By doing this pre-planning, we can shift all of these events into fun traditions that include exercise.

THIS LIFE PRACTICE IS POWERFUL.

If you intentionally follow the strategy we are about to look at below, you will find that you need very little grit or self-discipline to maintain exercise during holidays and big annual events. Your active lifestyle will have a life of its own. If you follow this strategy, you will become one of the amazing few who are able to exercise throughout holidays and events.

Here are a few examples of holidays, events, or other big items that typically get in the way of exercise. Next to each event, I listed an idea of what I could do that day as a new exercise tradition.

- **Thanksgiving:** *Include a walk after the meal.*

- **Vacation:** *Pick a location that will encourage you to relax AND exercise.*

- **Child's Birthday:** *Encourage them to choose active games, and then join in the fun.*

- **Long Travel Day:** *Carve out time the day before to get in a great workout. Plan ahead and protect the time.*

- **Corporate Retreat:** *Decide to go for a walk before dinner or add a couple of short walks during breaks.*

In a previous lesson, we looked at the concept of having a multi-year approach for exercising during holidays. Now let's begin to practice this concept in your life. It's easy to implement, but it does require a commitment. Let's unpack this strategy here.

The two-year strategy takes you through three rounds of any given holiday, vacation, or annual event.

Year #1—Create a Plan and Do It
You intentionally start a new active lifestyle tradition and invite a few friends to join.

Year #2—Adjust and Repeat
Your friends are HOPING you will do something similar—and you will!

Year #3—Magic Happens
Your friends are EXPECTING you to do it again. It is the NEW NORMAL.

Here's an example of how this strategy plays out.
For this example, we will use Labor Day weekend, a major three-day weekend that traditionally marks the unofficial end of summer in the United States. It is also a time when many people do everything BUT exercise.

Year #1—Create a Plan and Do It
What activity do you want to do on this day?

> **Example:** *This Labor Day weekend, you decide your festivities will include hiking. You've never done this before. You invite friends to join you. Some of your current friends decline because they're just not into it, and you have to reach a little further to find friends to join you. You are committed to hiking regardless of whether you get a big group to join you.*

How will this plan play out for you?

> **Example:** *When Labor Day weekend arrives, you go on that hike you planned. You're getting to know a new friend, or your old friends have joined, and you're having a great time on the hike. Exercise brings people together and helps everyone feel good. You feel good that you were able to accomplish this goal.*

....

Year #2—Adjust and Repeat

What will the following year look like?

> **Example:** *Fast forward to a year later. It's Labor Day weekend again, and now your friends who had a great time with you a year ago are HOPING you'll do something similar again. Congratulations, you have become the leader of this new tradition!*

....

BUT WAIT—THERE'S MORE!

(Cheesy, I know. I just couldn't resist.)

Year #3—Magic Happens

Fast forward to the third year. You have done your hiking tradition for two years and are now headed toward year number three. Your friends are not just hoping you'll plan something similar, they are EXPECTING it will happen. You have finally reached the nirvana of "active lifestyle as a normal way of life!"

Why This Is Important to You: Small changes create big magic.

You can make life changes overnight, but you'll need a couple of years to solidify them. When you own your annual events, holidays, and obligations and incorporate exercise into them, you have set up powerful traditions that grow into a life of their own. No more grit, no more drudgery, no more massive doses of self-discipline needed. The ship is now sailing itself, and you're finally along for the ride!

This type of long-term thinking is an amazingly powerful tool that will help you take control of the direction of your life. You have to think ahead and plan something you will enjoy year after year.

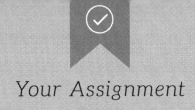

Your Assignment

It's your turn to think through one of your annual events or holidays and create a plan to shake it up.

Pick ONE event in your year and make a new plan for that date that includes activity or exercise rather than sedentary sitting and eating all day.

In the next lesson, you will make a plan for your entire year. For today, let's warm up with this one exercise.

IT'S YOUR TURN; LET'S DO THIS!

Pick ONE annual event, holiday, or vacation from your life and follow the steps below.

My annual holiday or event: _____

On this holiday or event, what exercise plan are you going to follow? Write your plan here.

Are there any barriers to success that you need to plan for ahead of the event?

That was a good practice round. In the coming lesson, we are going to work through this exercise for an entire year's worth of holidays and events.

HOLIDAYS AND EVENTS

In the previous lesson, you practiced planning ahead for a holiday or other annual event. In this lesson, the rubber meets the road, and you are going to look at an entire year of your holidays, birthdays, and other annual events.

When it comes to holidays and other annual events, being proactive is your best ally. You will look at an entire year and list all of the holidays, birthdays, and other events that could hinder your progress. You will work through an entire year listing each item and then brainstorming a solution for each and every item. This process involves a fair amount of effort, so give yourself a solid hour to work through it.

LOOK AHEAD. STAY AHEAD. IT'S THE EASIEST PATH.

Here's a list of common holidays and annual events that can get in the way of exercise.

UNITED STATES EVENTS AND HOLIDAYS

ALL YEAR
Birthdays
Anniversaries
Corporate Events
Retreats
Vacations
Kids' Events

JANUARY
New Year's Day
Martin Luther King Jr. Day

FEBRUARY
Groundhog Day
Super Bowl Sunday
Lincoln's Birthday
Valentine's Day
Ash Wednesday
Presidents' Day
Mid-Winter Break

MARCH
Daylight Savings Starts

APRIL
Easter
Spring Break
Tax Day

MAY
Cinco de Mayo
Mother's Day
Armed Forces Day
Memorial Day Weekend

JUNE
Father's Day

JULY
Independence Day
Summer vacations
Summer events

AUGUST
Summer vacations
Summer events

SEPTEMBER
Labor Day Weekend
School Starts

OCTOBER
Columbus/Indigenous People's Day
Halloween

NOVEMBER
Daylight Savings Ends
Veterans Day
Thanksgiving
Black Friday

DECEMBER
There are too many here to list; include your holidays observed plus holiday events and New Year's Eve.

If you add it all up, there is over a month's worth of exercise that can easily get lost with all of these days that we tend to dismiss as special exceptions. Wow! No wonder consistent exercise is so difficult! Even if you have an easy schedule, a low-stress job, and minimal obligations, you are still constantly bombarded with all kinds of other events that get in the way of exercise! This is why planning ahead for all of these is so critically important. Planning ahead and creating a new routine for annual events is a powerful way to put yourself back into the driver's seat of your life.

Creating a plan for the month ahead has really helped me stay on track. When I'm able to visualize how I can stay active even when I have a lot going on in my life, I know I'll be able to follow through. Tip: Don't just think through what you're going to do—make sure you write it down! **–Jason**

Your Assignment

PART ONE: *Make your plan*

In Appendix B of this book, you will find a full calendar set of pages that look like this one. Fill out all of the twelve monthly pages with all of your holidays, vacations, and any other events that happen annually in your life. For each and every item, think about how you can adjust that event so that it can include exercise you enjoy.

15

JANUARY

PLAN TO SUCCEED!

EVENTS & HOLIDAYS	EXERCISE PLAN

PART TWO: *Calendar it*

I know you won't be carrying this book with you every day for the next year, so let's make sure your work doesn't get lost.

Your task: Go to your personal calendar now and create a reminder for you to look at this plan on the first day of each month. Your calendar reminder could look something like this.

> **FIRST OF EVERY MONTH:**
> **"REVIEW COUCH TO ACTIVE PLAN."**

Put this recurring reminder on your calendar *right now!*

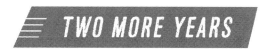

TWO MORE YEARS

If we stopped here, you would risk falling back into your old sedentary habits.

YOU ARE NOT GOING TO LET THIS HAPPEN.

Your friends and family are probably beginning to notice a change in you, but they have no idea how long this change is going to last. If they think about the work you've accomplished so far, they may be curious as to whether this change is going to last.

The work you do over the next two years is THE KEY to your continued success. It's this work that will make your active lifestyle completely gel into a normal way of life for you.

Introducing the COUCH to ACTIVE Two-Year plan.

Here's how the two-year plan works. For the next two years, you will complete these three simple tasks on the first day of each month. That's right—you are going to repeat this exercise every month for two full years.

1. **Review this COUCH to ACTIVE book.**

    Decide which ONE life practice you will continue to improve in the upcoming month. Appendix D includes a condensed list of the main life practices covered in the book.

2. **Review your WHY.**

    It's important that you stay crystal clear on WHY you are making this change in your life. Each month, you will remind yourself of WHY this is important to you. Your WHY may stay the same month after month or change over time. What's most important is that you are brutally honest with yourself and dig deep.

3. **Plan Ahead.**

    Open your calendar and look at the month in front of you. Mark out any holidays or any other big events that might get in the way, such as birthdays, vacations, or big projects at work. For each big event on your calendar, write down how you will get in exercise on that day. Create a plan now, and it will help you follow through when the day arises. Don't skip these workouts!

Your Assignment

PART ONE: *Calendar reminders*

Go into your calendar and double-check that the first of the month calendar reminders you created from the previous lesson are still there. You should have reminders in place for a full two years. Update these reminders to include the instructions in part two of your assignment below.

PART TWO: *First-of-the-month work*

On the first day of each month for the next two years, work through the three parts of the two-year plan.

1. Review this COUCH to ACTIVE book. Which life practice will you focus on this month? (You can find the life practice list in Appendix D in the back of this book.)

2. WHY is having an active lifestyle important to you today?

3. Plan Ahead: Look at your calendar for the upcoming month and plan for all events such as holidays, birthdays, and anniversaries that may normally get in the way of exercise. Make your exercise plan for each of these days. Tip: It is okay to have your plan include a longer workout on the day BEFORE a holiday.

👍 **PRO TIP:** If you prefer to have a workbook to complete, COUCH to ACTIVE has a Two-Year Workbook published.
For more information, go to www.couchtoactive.com

ESCAPE A SETBACK

What will you do if you have a setback? It's no secret that life is crazy-as-bananas. You will face unexpected barriers, new challenges, and big life events. Any one of these could cause a setback. This lesson walks you through a quick and effective tool to jumpstart your mindset back to an active lifestyle.

Mindset is critically important in maintaining your active lifestyle. Focus on who you have become and repeat to yourself, "I am active." Don't let your mind wander back to the valley of sadness where you begin to doubt your progress.

I AM ACTIVE!

The great thing about this exercise is that you can complete it right where you are during a setback—from your couch!

In the following assignment, you are going to walk through a series of questions that are designed to help you escape a setback. During this exercise dig deep and find your renewed energy and commitment to your active lifestyle.

Take your time and dig deep.
Your active lifestyle is worth it.
You are worth it.
You are worthy.

I've tried to get and stay active many times in my life...and I've failed a whole bunch of times, too. In the past, I would let my setbacks get the best of me. This time, I chose to stay focused and remind myself that a setback doesn't have power over me. It won't ruin my new habits forever, and I can get back in the rhythm. **–Zoe**

Your Assignment

Complete this anytime you have a setback.

I know that most of you are not in the middle of a setback, so you're going to need to use your imagination when practicing this assignment today. Pretend you are having a setback sometime in the future, and use this opportunity to become familiar with the exercise.

Below is a list of questions you are going to work through. It is your choice if you write your answers on paper or just think them through. Do what will give you the best results. If you normally talk out loud to process information, then talk away!

Dig deep and find your renewed energy for your active lifestyle.

MINDSET EXERCISE: ESCAPE A SETBACK

1. Think about when you are your best at living an active lifestyle. What does it look like? How does it feel?

2. What is the disconnect between how you are currently using your time and this vision?

3. How will you feel when you get back into your active lifestyle?

4. What if you DO get back to your active lifestyle right now? What will your life look like one year from today?

5. What if you DON'T and you continue to slide backwards? What will your life look like one year from today?

6. What barriers do you need to overcome to get back on track?

7. Who in your life will benefit from you getting back on track? How will those people benefit?

8. On a scale of 1-10, how confident are you that you will succeed?

9. What can you do this week to increase your chances of success?

10. What excuses are coming up for you right now that you need to stop using?

11. Are there any areas where you need to show yourself compassion? Are you being too tough on yourself, or are you setting unrealistic expectations?

12. Remind yourself that you HAVE made great progress. Think of the successes you have accomplished so far. What helped you succeed?

13. Remind yourself that massive frustration is good. It means you haven't given up and you are still motivated to make progress.

14. Think of your loved ones. Remind yourself that they do want you to be healthy, but they might not know how to express their feelings to you.

15. What types of exercise do you enjoy most? When can you do this exercise next?

16. Remind yourself: "I am worthy of a healthy life, which means I am worthy of an active lifestyle. I AM WORTHY." Repeat this over and over until you believe it.

"I am worthy. This will never change."

MINDSET: REVISIT THIS NON-NEGOTIABLE PASSAGE.

My body needs exercise.
My body will always need exercise.
This will never change.
It's not negotiable, it's science.

NEXT STEP: MAKE A PLAN

Here are your next action items. Complete them right now.

1. Right now, plan a specific time to do the exercise you enjoy.

2. Review the life practices that are listed in Appendix D of this book.

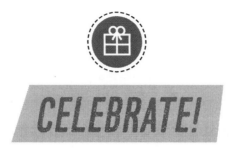

WEEK EIGHT

Celebrate the new you!

Exercise:

Go to Appendix C of this book and complete your exercise plans for Week 8.

Schedule your exercise plans into your calendar.

Lessons:

You = Rock star!

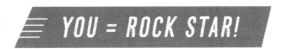

YOU = ROCK STAR!

That's right—you are a rock star!

Consider this. Only 21% of adults in the United States reach the minimum exercise levels recommended by the Centers for Disease Control. That's right—only 1 in 5 adults gets the minimum exercise needed. Congratulations, you are now part of the top 21%. Compared to 80% of adults in the United States, you are rocking it!

NOT CONVINCED YOU ARE ROCKING IT? HANG TIGHT WHILE I GET UP ON MY SOAPBOX FOR A FEW MINUTES . . . .

Until our whole nation becomes more active, you are going to be a trailblazer. You are now a leader in the community of exercise. By being part of the top 21% in the United States, like it or not, you are a role model. It's hard work to lead this trend when the majority of people around you are not yet exercising like you are. My dream is that someday these numbers will reverse and the majority of adults will join the ranks of those who exercise. It will be so much easier for all of us when this shift happens!

So celebrate! Laugh! Cheer on those who are rocking it with you.

And if that's not enough to convince you, please let me continue . . . .

YOU HAVE COVERED SO MUCH GROUND.

The Basics: You are now crystal clear on the baseline for exercise and what is non-negotiable. You've connected with your doctor and are staying injury-free. You understand better than most that exercise is not negotiable and that consistent exercise is not normal for our nation. You are not normal—in a very good way!

YOU'RE ROCKING IT IN A NEW WAY!

Reaching Out: You now have tools to empower you to turn on the support of your friends and family in pursuit of your active lifestyle. You are working on making bridges with them. You are not judgmental of their sedentary lives because you know you were there not long ago, and you understand the path to getting active is much more than just needing more grit or self-discipline. You are relentlessly pursuing exercise you find fun, and you are letting go of exercise you dread.

YOU'RE ROCKING IT FOR YOUR FRIENDS!

Barriers: You now see your barriers more clearly than ever, and you're seeing which barriers you can break and which barriers you can't change today. You know how to take new barriers that come your way and quickly decide whether you are going to break the barrier or work with it. You are not letting your jiggly body get in the way of going out and being active. Instead, you are being brave and thereby letting others know it's safe for them to also be brave and join you.

YOU ARE LOOKING YOUR BARRIERS STRAIGHT IN THE EYE AND ROCKING IT!

Owning It: You are owning your success, owning your excuses, owning your opinions, owning your heart, and owning your time. You embrace the fact that life is crazy-as-bananas. You wouldn't want a boring life! Most importantly, you are recognizing when you need healing, and you are resourceful in finding ways to heal. You no longer wait for permission to own your life. It's yours to live.

YOU ARE ROCKING YOUR DESTINY!

Radical Change: You are feeling more empowered to make radical changes in your life. You are seeing the difference between truly being stuck and making big excuses. When you see a barrier that cannot change right away, you practice patience and self-compassion. You are mustering up massive courage so you can face the biggest changes needed.

YOU ARE ROCKING YOUR WORLD!

Two-Year Plan: You now have a framework to continue all of this great progress. You are on the path with a clear direction to cement these changes and make them part of your new normal. This long-term progress is what will make the magic happen and solidify your new active lifestyle.

YOU'RE ROCKING YOUR LONG-TERM SUCCESS!

SO YES, THAT'S RIGHT. YOU = ROCK STAR!

Congratulations and big hugs to you, my new friend.

Welcome to your new life.

If we haven't met in person, I hope to someday. It's a small world we share.

This journey has been my humble honor.

Lyn Lindbergh
Your Bad Couch Guru

PS. Above all, have compassion for yourself and always stay true to living a life you love!

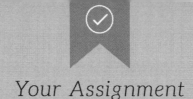

Your Assignment

YOU ARE A ROCK STAR!

That's right—you are rocking it more than you realize. This final assignment is meant to help you recognize the progress you have made and leave you feeling proud of where you are.

PART ONE: *Star chart*

Appendix D contains a list of life practices you learned in this book. Put a star next to each one that you have either made progress in or feel you currently do well. Each time you review the list, add a star next to any additional items where you are making great progress.

THE BASICS

LIFE PRACTICES

- No more exercise I hate. ☆
- Live a life I love. ☆
- Challenge what is normal.
- I am a human who needs exercise. ☆
- I call my doctor when needed.
- I stay injury-free. ☆
- I will remember to exercise.
- Slow and steady progress—the turtle wins!
- Clean out my toxic social media. ☆

PART TWO: *Celebrate*

Congratulations! Your final assignment is to celebrate your accomplishment. DON'T SKIP YOUR CELEBRATION! Ask yourself right now, "what kind of celebration would make me smile?"

It's hard to believe we have come to the end of the program. Whew! I wish you all the best in your crazy-as-bananas life!

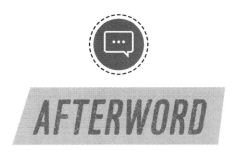

AFTERWORD

At this very moment, I am finishing the manuscript for this book from my hotel room. I am at the tail end of having just spent another week attending a major fitness convention. As I walked through the vendor booths of the convention hall, I was left with a looming feeling that sadly, the marketing of most exercise and fitness companies is still completely off-target. I was bombarded by air-brushed bikini bodies, sweaty six-pack abs, and offers to pour your paycheck into the next magic potion, lotion, and pill. It quite literally makes me sick to my stomach. Yesterday afternoon, I left the convention hall early and went back to my hotel room to chillax and decompress from it all.

This week, I also attended fitness demonstration classes at the convention and heard premiere instructors actually say these exact words:

"Girls, we're going to get rid of the junk in your trunk!"

"Let's get our bikini bodies on!"

"Twerk it baby, twerk it!"

"This will fix your flat butt!"

"If it hurts your joints, that's normal."

In this era of the Me Too movement and big scientific data, we should all know better. No wonder most of the population polarizes against this. I do, too.

There is a message of hope. I'm seeing a steady shift in the right direction. There is a lot of momentum headed toward exercise as a lifestyle, exercise as a fun activity, exercise as a way to build community, and exercise as a way to enhance your life today. I am optimistic this improvement will continue because you are now part of this movement. Thank you!

NO MORE EXERCISE WE HATE!

YOU = ACTIVE!

EXERCISE PLAN EXAMPLES

Exercise Plan 1

I HATE EXERCISING, BUT MY DOCTOR IS MAKING ME DO THIS.

You hate exercise, but fear for your health. I get it. This is a very good reason to start exercising, but it's a terrible way to stay motivated to continue with what you start. I want you to first read the chapter titled "Make it Fun." Figuring out how to enjoy exercise is going to be key to your success. Then carefully study the entire first section of the book titled "The Basics." I can pretty much guarantee that if you jump full on into a tough exercise program, you will get injured. Don't make this mistake. Instead, spend the next four to six months very slowly building up the exercises you enjoy. Exercise is not a punishment, and it can become a joy. I will help you get there.

MY EXERCISE

Create your own exercise plan for the week.

WEEK OF ___ / ___ / ___

TYPE/DAY	EXERCISE	DONE
♡ SUN	Rest and stretch.	✓
♡ MON	Exercises my doctor prescribed.	✓
⫩ TUE	Exercise I think might be fun.	✓
♡ WED	Exercises my doctor prescribed.	✓
⫩ THU	Exercise I think might be fun.	✓
♡ FRI	Makeup day for exercise I missed.	✓
♡ SAT	A walk that is five minutes longer than normal.	✓

Exercise Plan 2

MY DRIVER'S LICENSE SAYS I'M 55, BUT I'LL BE 30 FOREVER.

Let's face it—we are middle-aged, but in denial. Keep on rocking it! I have so much respect for people who relentlessly pursue the rebellion against gravity! You are young at heart and always will be. Let's keep that spirit shining.

Now, you already know this, but you must be committed to staying injury-free. If you have been sedentary and are just getting back to it, start with the plan below and spend the next four to six months slowly working your way up to more activity.

MY EXERCISE

Create your own exercise plan for the week.

WEEK OF ____ / ____ / ____

TYPE/DAY	EXERCISE	DONE
♡ SUN	Rest and stretch	✓
♡ MON	Cardio—Five minutes longer than what you normally do.	✓
⫞⫟ TUE	Weights—light and easy.	✓
♡ WED	Cardio—Five minutes longer than what you normally do.	✓
⫞⫟ THU	Weights—add a little more only if you are not sore from Tuesday.	✓
♡ FRI	Cardio—5 minutes longer than what you normally do.	✓
♡ SAT	Long slow walk, swim, or bike. Stay injury-free.	✓

Exercise Plan 3

HELP, I JUST GRADUATED COLLEGE AND AM COMPLETELY OUT OF SHAPE!

I hear you! You sacrificed a lot to get where you are today. When I graduated college, I couldn't run to the mailbox without getting winded. The exercise plan below is where you can begin if you are in your 20s or early 30s and have no pre-existing injuries. Over about four to six months, slowly add to this plan. The key is to not overdo it and slowly build. If you used to do sports back in your high school days, do NOT try to go right back to it. Injury-free is your fastest path to progress.

MY EXERCISE

Create your own exercise plan for the week.

WEEK OF ____ / ____ / ____

TYPE/DAY	EXERCISE	DONE
♡ SUN	*Rest and Stretch*	✓
♡ MON	*Walk/Jog 10 minutes*	✓
🏋 TUE	*Weights: Medium intensity, full body.*	✓
♡ WED	*Walk/Jog 15 minutes.*	✓
🏋 THU	*Weights: Medium intensity, full body.*	✓
♡ FRI	*Cardio—30 minutes easy.*	✓
♡ SAT	*Any exercise you enjoy for 60+ minutes.*	✓

Exercise Plan 4

I'M A CHRONIC MESS OF HEALTH ISSUES.

If this is you, compassion and patience is key. Avoid the trap of comparing yourself to anyone, including the person you were before you had these health issues. There is no such thing as a broken human, just people with very interesting lives they must live. Your barriers to exercise are very real and must be respected. Throughout this book, I am going to help you make peace with where you are today. Many fitness professionals are not well-trained in how to work with people who have unique health issues; you must advocate for yourself. Don't let anyone push you too fast, too soon. Use this plan as a place to start, then spend the next six months to two years slowly building strength as your body allows you to.

MY EXERCISE

Create your own exercise plan for the week.

WEEK OF ____ / ____ / ____

TYPE/DAY	EXERCISE	DONE
♡ SUN	*Rest and Stretch*	✓
♡ MON	*5 minutes of any exercise you can do.*	✓
⫘ TUE	*5 minutes of any exercise you can do.*	✓
♡ WED	*20 minutes of any exercise you can do.*	✓
⫘ THU	*Mindset work. Spend about 20 minutes breathing slowly and searching for inner peace about your health issues.*	✓
♡ FRI	*5 minutes of any exercise you can do.*	✓
♡ SAT	*30 minutes of anything you can do, no matter how small or simple it is.*	✓

Exercise Plan 5

THE BABY WON'T LET ME SLEEP!

If this is you, read the "Your Sleep" section of the chapter titled "Own It" (page 165). Take the Three-Day Sleep Test today. If you fail the sleep test, do not despair; just know this is an area to keep an eye on. Your children are your top priority, and I'm going to help you learn how to keep them your priority and make room for exercise in your life. My goal for you is not to give you a one-and-done solution, but to prepare you to handle the next 20 years of your life constantly shifting as your children grow. Use the exercise plan below as a baseline to begin, and then slowly add more exercise over the next four to six months.

MY EXERCISE

Create your own exercise plan for the week.

WEEK OF ____ /____ /____

TYPE/DAY	EXERCISE	DONE
♡ SUN	Take a nap (Seriously, take a nap if you can.)	✓
♡ MON	Playtime with baby!	✓
⫔ TUE	Eat healthy today and take another nap.	✓
♡ WED	Take baby for a long stroller walk.	✓
⫔ THU	Drink a ton of water today and take a nap.	✓
♡ FRI	Playtime with baby!	✓
♡ SAT	Take baby for a long stroller walk/jog.	✓

Exercise Plan 6

I HATE MY ASTHMA!

Asthma can be so frustrating, because you look generally healthy on the outside, but struggle with energy, and exercise can be scary. I hear you; it can be incredibly tough and lonely. People forget you are dealing with this silent disease, and your body won't keep up with your spirit. First and foremost, respect your lungs. You will have good days and bad, and sometimes it's impossible to predict how you will feel on any given day. When reading recommendations for exercise plans, remember that there is a high likelihood that you might need extra rest days between strenuous exercise. In this book, I spend time helping people with physical barriers learn how to make peace with where they are today. Use the exercise plan below as a starting place, and spend the next six months to two years slowly building your strength.

MY EXERCISE

Create your own exercise plan for the week.

WEEK OF _____ / _____ / _____

TYPE/DAY	EXERCISE	DONE
♡ SUN	Rest and Stretch	✓
♡ MON	Yoga, Pilates, or other non-cardio exercise.	✓
🏋 TUE	Walk only as long as you can without injuring your lungs.	✓
♡ WED	Weights, lightweight and easy, full body	✓
🏋 THU	Walk only as long as you can without injuring your lungs.	✓
♡ FRI	Mindset work. Spend about 20 minutes breathing slowly and searching for peace about your asthma.	✓
♡ SAT	Weights; slightly heavier if you are feeling good.	✓

Exercise Plan 7

I SERIOUSLY NEED TO LOSE 100 POUNDS.

If this is you, the concepts in this book will help you bring together exercise, food, and love of self to create a successful formula for major life change. If you're asking "what in the world does Lyn know about extreme weight loss?" I actually spend personal vacations at weight-loss resorts. I love the supportive environment and have incredible respect for people undergoing radical life change inside and out. It takes strength of character to undergo such a change. These weight-loss resorts are havens for me; I come home renewed and ready to jump back into my crazy-as-bananas life. For your exercise plan, start with what is listed below and then increase the duration and intensity over four to six months as your body allows you to do so injury-free.

MY EXERCISE

Create your own exercise plan for the week.

WEEK OF ____ /____ / ____

TYPE/DAY	EXERCISE	DONE
♡ SUN	Rest and Stretch	✓
♡ MON	Walk as long as you can without pain.	✓
⊣⊢ TUE	Do full body weights with very light weights.	✓
♡ WED	Swim as long as you can without pain.	✓
⊣⊢ THU	Do full body weights with slightly more weights.	✓
♡ FRI	Do anything that seems fun to you!	✓
♡ SAT	Enjoy nature. Hike as long as you can without pain.	✓

Exercise Plan 8

I DREAM OF COMPLETING A MARATHON.

Yes, you absolutely can train for a marathon. Don't let anyone discourage you. The runner's high is real, and it's an amazing thing to experience. Do stay committed to being injury-free. If you have been mostly sedentary, then start week one with the plan below and slowly build your strength. The number one mistake runners make is to do too much, too soon. Your fastest path to success is to stay steady and injury-free. Once you have built a base, then Google the Couch to 5K running plan for your next step. Best of luck, and send me a message when you cross your first finish line!

MY EXERCISE

Create your own exercise plan for the week.

WEEK OF ___ / ___ / ___

TYPE/DAY	EXERCISE	DONE
♡ SUN	Rest and Stretch.	✓
♡ MON	Walk/jog for as long as you can injury-free while maintaining a smile. This might be only 1 minute; that is perfectly fine.	✓
⫘ TUE	Light weights or yoga.	✓
♡ WED	Walk/jog for as long as you can injury-free while maintaining a smile. This might be only 1 minute; that is perfectly fine	✓
⫘ THU	Medium weights or yoga.	✓
♡ FRI	Walk/jog for as long as you can injury-free while maintaining a smile. This might be only 1 minute; that is perfectly fine.	✓
♡ SAT	Get into nature and go for a longer hike, preferably with hills.	✓

Exercise Plan 9

I'M ALREADY IN GREAT SHAPE.

If you are already in great shape, then why are you reading this book?

All right, I know that all of us can benefit from exercise motivation, even myself. On this plan, we are going to get your Vo2Max to increase. By following a plan similar to the one on the next page, your heart and lungs will begin to process oxygen more efficiently. This translates to feeling stronger and happier every day of your life. It means you will live a life with a daily rush of endorphins that will make it easier for you to smile every single day. Isn't that a great way to live? Use a plan similar to this one, and aim for a total of five to six hours of exercise each week. Consistency is key.

Just because you are in great shape doesn't mean exercising consistently comes easy for you and it doesn't automatically mean you have a healthy approach to exercise. Are you comparing yourself to others in an unhealthy way? Are holding yourself to a ridiculous standard that is causing you to be stressed out and highly self-critical? We are going to look at this together.

Throughout this book, you will also experience how to change the dialogue on exercise motivation. There are a lot of reasons why our status quo on exercise motivation is failing us, and most of the fitness industry is blind to the real reasons most of us don't get our tennis shoes on. Your compassion for others is going to grow, and you'll learn how to make exercise a part of your life without requiring so much grit and self-discipline. Your friends or clients will love the fact that you "get it" and can help them right where they are today.

MY EXERCISE

Create your own exercise plan for the week.

WEEK OF ___ / ___ / ___

TYPE/DAY	EXERCISE	DONE
♡ SUN	*30 minutes of easy walking/jogging.*	✓
♡ MON	*30 minutes of weight-bearing exercises.*	✓
⫶⊞⫶ TUE	*30 minutes of intervals plus 30 minutes of cardio.*	✓
♡ WED	*30 minutes of weight-bearing exercises.*	✓
⫶⊞⫶ THU	*30 minutes of easy cardio such as a walk.*	✓
♡ FRI	*30 minutes of intervals, plus 30 minutes of cardio.*	✓
♡ SAT	*90+ minutes of any exercise you enjoy.*	✓

APPENDICES

MINIMUM EXERCISE (A)

Are you exercising enough to stave off preventable disease?
There are so many experts out there telling you what you should be doing
for exercise that it can be difficult to know who is right.

The Centers for Disease Control have published physical activity recommendations. The good news is that their recommendations are incredibly flexible. They recognize that there are many different ways to exercise and that it's all about simply moving your body.

This is the minimum baseline that you should work to achieve each week. If this seems like a lot of exercise for you, then it's important to start where you are and gradually work up to this level of exercise. Give yourself a full four to six months to reach this level, and if you have special health concerns, it might take you much longer to achieve this level. It's important to respect where your body is today and give it time to adjust to its new normal.

Moderate-Intensity Aerobic Examples
Brisk walk, swimming, water aerobics, dancing, kick-boxing, biking, hiking, gardening, Duck Duck Goose, yard work, water skiing, chasing kids, power walk the mall, stairs, volleyball, kayaking, surfing, kick ball, tennis.

Muscle-Strengthening Examples
Weights, yoga, Pilates, pull ups, push ups, abdominals, squats, calf raises, leg extensions, bicep curls, butterfly press, back extension, modified planks.

For all exercise programs, the rule of thumb is this: move your body as much as possible while staying injury-free. Do not feel pressured to follow a dogmatic and rigid routine. It is common for people to begin exercising and neglect the muscle-strengthening work. It is important to find a way to keep these integrated into your routine.

Here is the CDC's basic recommendation for adults:

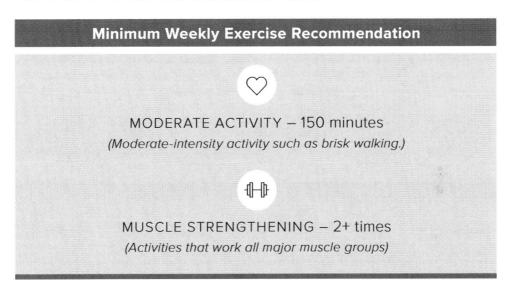

Minimum Weekly Exercise Recommendation

MODERATE ACTIVITY — 150 minutes
(Moderate-intensity activity such as brisk walking.)

MUSCLE STRENGTHENING — 2+ times
(Activities that work all major muscle groups)

If you are training for a specific event or outcome, such as completing a 5K race, then you will need to use exercise plans specific to those goals. But for general health and well-being, simply keep the entire body moving.

MONTHLY EXERCISE GUIDE (B)

Here is an example of how you can fit the minimum exercise recommendations into a month of exercise. This is just one example of many possibilities designed to help you see how a month of exercise could play out in your life. It's a great place to start.

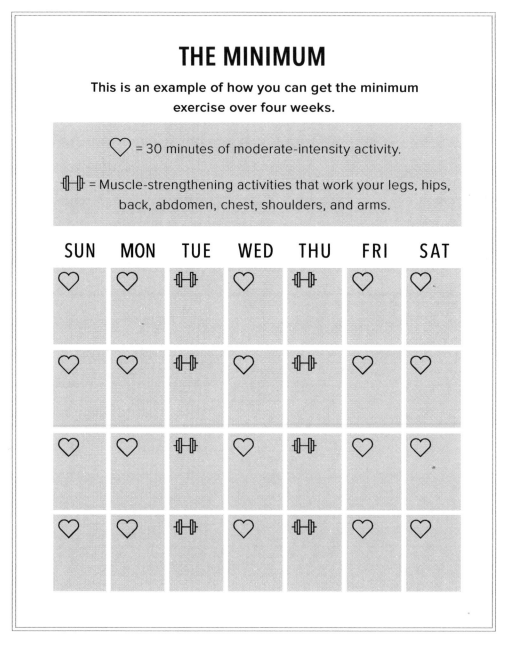

THE MINIMUM

This is an example of how you can get the minimum exercise over four weeks.

♡ = 30 minutes of moderate-intensity activity.

⫴ = Muscle-strengthening activities that work your legs, hips, back, abdomen, chest, shoulders, and arms.

SUN	MON	TUE	WED	THU	FRI	SAT
♡	♡	⫴	♡	⫴	♡	♡
♡	♡	⫴	♡	⫴	♡	♡
♡	♡	⫴	♡	⫴	♡	♡
♡	♡	⫴	♡	⫴	♡	♡

MONTHLY EXERCISE

Use these twelve planner sheets when you reach the lesson titled "Holidays and Events." Your directions are in the assignment of that lesson.

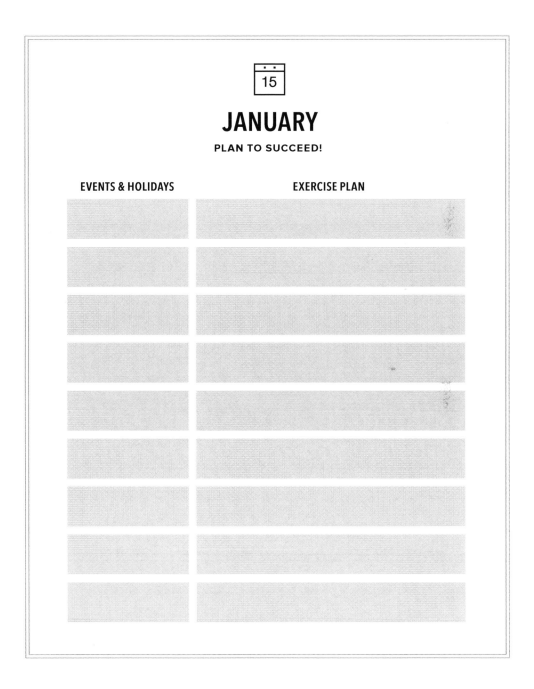

JANUARY
PLAN TO SUCCEED!

EVENTS & HOLIDAYS	EXERCISE PLAN

15

FEBRUARY

PLAN TO SUCCEED!

EVENTS & HOLIDAYS	EXERCISE PLAN

📅 15

MARCH

PLAN TO SUCCEED!

EVENTS & HOLIDAYS   **EXERCISE PLAN**

APRIL

PLAN TO SUCCEED!

EVENTS & HOLIDAYS	EXERCISE PLAN

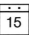

MAY

PLAN TO SUCCEED!

EVENTS & HOLIDAYS	EXERCISE PLAN

15

JUNE

PLAN TO SUCCEED!

EVENTS & HOLIDAYS	EXERCISE PLAN

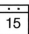

JULY

PLAN TO SUCCEED!

EVENTS & HOLIDAYS	EXERCISE PLAN

15

AUGUST

PLAN TO SUCCEED!

EVENTS & HOLIDAYS	EXERCISE PLAN

15

SEPTEMBER

PLAN TO SUCCEED!

EVENTS & HOLIDAYS	EXERCISE PLAN

15

OCTOBER

PLAN TO SUCCEED!

EVENTS & HOLIDAYS	EXERCISE PLAN

15

NOVEMBER

PLAN TO SUCCEED!

EVENTS & HOLIDAYS	EXERCISE PLAN

15

DECEMBER

PLAN TO SUCCEED!

EVENTS & HOLIDAYS	EXERCISE PLAN

WEEKLY EXERCISE PLANS (C)

Use these blank worksheets to help you plan your exercise for each week as you work through the COUCH to ACTIVE program. Use the images of the hearts and weights to remind you to mix up the type of exercise you do throughout the week.

MY EXERCISE

Create your own exercise plan for the week.

WEEK OF ____ / ____ / ____

TYPE/DAY	EXERCISE	DONE
♡ SUN		✓
♡ MON		✓
⫴ TUE		✓
♡ WED		✓
⫴ THU		✓
♡ FRI		✓
♡ SAT		✓

MY EXERCISE

Create your own exercise plan for the week.

WEEK OF ___ /___ /___

TYPE/DAY	EXERCISE	DONE
♡ SUN		✓
♡ MON		✓
⫟ TUE		✓
♡ WED		✓
⫟ THU		✓
♡ FRI		✓
♡ SAT		✓

MY EXERCISE

Create your own exercise plan for the week.

WEEK OF ___ /___ /___

TYPE/DAY	EXERCISE	DONE
♡ SUN		✓
♡ MON		✓
⫟ TUE		✓
♡ WED		✓
⫟ THU		✓
♡ FRI		✓
♡ SAT		✓

MY EXERCISE

Create your own exercise plan for the week.

WEEK OF ___ /___ / ___

TYPE/DAY	EXERCISE	DONE
♡ SUN		⊘
♡ MON		⊘
⫯⫯ TUE		⊘
♡ WED		⊘
⫯⫯ THU		⊘
♡ FRI		⊘
♡ SAT		⊘

MY EXERCISE

Create your own exercise plan for the week.

WEEK OF ___ /___ / ___

TYPE/DAY	EXERCISE	DONE
♡ SUN		⊘
♡ MON		⊘
⫯⫯ TUE		⊘
♡ WED		⊘
⫯⫯ THU		⊘
♡ FRI		⊘
♡ SAT		⊘

MY EXERCISE

Create your own exercise plan for the week.

WEEK OF ___ /___ / ___

TYPE/DAY	EXERCISE	DONE
♡ SUN		✓
♡ MON		✓
⫤ TUE		✓
♡ WED		✓
⫤ THU		✓
♡ FRI		✓
♡ SAT		✓

MY EXERCISE

Create your own exercise plan for the week.

WEEK OF ___ /___ / ___

TYPE/DAY	EXERCISE	DONE
♡ SUN		✓
♡ MON		✓
⫤ TUE		✓
♡ WED		✓
⫤ THU		✓
♡ FRI		✓
♡ SAT		✓

MY EXERCISE

Create your own exercise plan for the week.

WEEK OF ____ /____ / ____

TYPE/DAY	EXERCISE	DONE
♡ SUN		✓
♡ MON		✓
⫟ TUE		✓
♡ WED		✓
⫟ THU		✓
♡ FRI		✓
♡ SAT		✓

MY EXERCISE

Create your own exercise plan for the week.

WEEK OF ____ /____ / ____

TYPE/DAY	EXERCISE	DONE
♡ SUN		✓
♡ MON		✓
⫟ TUE		✓
♡ WED		✓
⫟ THU		✓
♡ FRI		✓
♡ SAT		✓

LIFE PRACTICES (D)

The following pages highlight the key life practices from this book. On the first day of each month, review the lists below and reflect on how you have succeeded and what you can do differently in the coming weeks.

MEMORIZE THIS!

MY BODY NEEDS EXERCISE.

MY BODY WILL ALWAYS NEED EXERCISE.

THIS WILL NEVER CHANGE.

IT'S NOT NEGOTIABLE, IT'S SCIENCE!

THE BASICS

No more exercise I hate.

I aim to live a life I love.

I challenge what is normal.

I am a human who needs to exercise.

I call my doctor when needed.

I stay injury-free.

I remember to exercise.

I use slow and steady progress as my key to success.

I monitor and clean out toxic social media.

REACH OUT

I talk to others about the importance of my active lifestyle.

I look my loved ones in the eyes and with love let them know that I am now living an active lifestyle; this will not change.

I am the first to reach out to others to plan exercise activities. I don't worry about always being the planner.

I know my friends may not notice my change right away. This is okay.

I thank the people who support me.

I relentlessly pursue figuring out how to make exercise fun.

BARRIERS

I list my barriers to exercise to help me clearly see solutions.

When I'm frustrated or overwhelmed, I slow down and give myself compassion.

I use walking as a tool to clear my mind to help me see solutions.

I start by breaking the barriers that I can influence today.

My body may jiggle more than I want it to, but I don't let that stop me.

I ignore the naysayers in my life.

I look for mini-solutions to exercise and then jump on the opportunities.

I am brave and try all kinds of exercise.

I make some of my exercise impossible to flake.

BARRIER ZONES

I get crystal clear on which barriers are the easiest to break.

OWN IT

I own my success.

My opinions matter; I have strong opinions about the importance of exercise.

The people closest to my heart want me to be healthy.

I own my time; really, I do own my time.

My life is crazy, and that's okay.

When I need healing, I am resourceful, and I find the tools and time.

Sleep is not only good for my body, but it also helps my brain to find solutions.

RADICAL CHANGE

I am empowered to make radical changes in my life.

When I'm frustrated, I pause and ask myself, "Am I really stuck? Or do I need to be brave?"

Some of my barriers are here to stay. This is okay.

Sometimes I need to be massively brave and make a big step in a new direction.

Other times, I need to carefully research the right solution.

Other times, I need to breathe and show myself compassion.

I never let myself stay stuck for too long.

I am worthy.

TWO YEARS

I blinked and the last two years flew by.

I will blink and the next two years will also fly by.

I am making the most of the next two years to dial in my new active lifestyle.

Life will always be changing, and my active lifestyle will always be adjusting to match.

I don't expect life to be perfect.

I always strive to improve.

I focus on living a life I love.

MY LIST

Do you have any unique life practices? Write them here.

COUCH TO ACTIVE RESOURCES

The COUCH to ACTIVE Program with Lyn

Working with a coach can be the difference between achieving your goals and falling short. If you have had this book for several months and still haven't made it through the entire program, then working with me might be exactly what you need. Learn more at www.couchtoactive.com/program.

COUCH to ACTIVE Private Workshops

Do you have a group that would benefit from working through this program together? I host workshops for groups of all sizes. Contact me through www.couchtoactive.com/workshops

Lyn as Your Keynote

Need a memorable and inspiring keynote speaker? In my corporate training experience, I saw the full range of speakers—from the excellent to those who committed murder by PowerPoint. I can deliver a customized keynote that will inspire your team to action. The concepts in this program reach so much further than simply exercise; I can show your team how to apply these principles to everything from sales to personal relationships to management. Contact me through www.couchtoactive.com/hire

Book Clubs

Thinking of sipping wine with a group of friends while enjoying this book? I read your mind! Check out my leader's guide for book clubs. www.couchtoactive.com/bookclubs

COUCH to ACTIVE for Health and Fitness Professionals

The reason people don't return to your gym or studio usually has nothing to do with how amazing your program is and everything to do with the lessons in this book. Learn more about how you can use the concepts of COUCH to ACTIVE to help your clients consistently return to you. www.couchtoactive.com/fitpro

The Two-Year Workbook

Sometimes having a printed version is the easiest way to go. The work described in the chapter about Your Next Two Years is already published in a Two-Year Workbook. Learn more about this workbook and where to purchase it at www.couchtoactive.com/twoyears

The COUCH to ACTIVE Podcast

When your hands are tied, a podcast could be exactly what you need to keep momentum going. Subscribe to Lyn Lindbergh's podcast titled COUCH to ACTIVE. www.couchtoactive.com/podcast

NOTES

NOTES

NOTES

NOTES

NOTES

NOTES

NOTES

NOTES